Overcoming I

WINDY DRYDEN was born in London in 195_ _____ ____ ___ ___
therapy and counselling for over 30 years, and is the author or editor of
over 160 books, including *How to Accept Yourself* (Sheldon Press, 1999)
and *Overcoming Envy* (Sheldon Press, 2002). Dr Dryden is Professor of
Psychotherapeutic Studies at Goldsmiths College, University of London.

Overcoming Common Problems Series

Selected titles

A full list of titles is available from Sheldon Press,
36 Causton Street, London SW1P 4ST and on our website at
www.sheldonpress.co.uk

The Assertiveness Handbook
Mary Hartley

Cataract: What You Need to Know
Mark Watts

Cider Vinegar
Margaret Hills

Coping Successfully with Period Problems
Mary-Claire Mason

Age-related Memory Loss
Dr Tom Smith

Coping with Blushing
Professor Robert Edelmann

Coping with Bowel Cancer
Dr Tom Smith

Coping with Brain Injury
Maggie Rich

Coping with Candida
Shirley Trickett

Coping with Chemotherapy
Dr Terry Priestman

Coping with Gout
Christine Craggs-Hinton

Coping with Hearing Loss
Christine Craggs-Hinton

Coping with Heartburn and Reflux
Dr Tom Smith

Coping with Macular Degeneration
Dr Patricia Gilbert

Coping with Polycystic Ovary Syndrome
Christine Craggs-Hinton

Coping with Postnatal Depression
Sandra L. Wheatley

Depressive Illness
Dr Tim Cantopher

Helping Children Cope with Anxiety
Jill Eckersley

How to Approach Death
Julia Tugendhat

How to Be a Healthy Weight
Philippa Pigache

How to Keep Cholesterol in Check
Dr Robert Povey

How to Make Life Happen
Gladeana McMahon

How to Succeed in Psychometric Tests
David Cohen

How to Talk to Your Child
Penny Oates

Living with Heart Failure
Susan Elliot-Wright

Living with Autism
Fiona Marshall

Living with Fibromyalgia
Christine Craggs-Hinton

Living with a Seriously Ill Child
Dr Jan Aldridge

Living with Loss and Grief
Julia Tugendhat

Living with Rheumatoid Arthritis
Philippa Pigache

Losing a Child
Linda Hurcombe

Overcoming Hurt
Dr Windy Dryden

Simplify Your Life
Naomi Saunders

The Depression Diet Book
Theresa Cheung

The Multiple Sclerosis Diet Book
Tessa Buckley

The PMS Handbook
Theresa Cheung

The Thinking Person's Guide to Happiness
Ruth Searle

The Traveller's Good Health Guide
Dr Ted Lankester

Treat Your Own Knees
Jim Johnson

Treating Arthritis – The Drug-free Way
Margaret Hills

Overcoming Common Problems

Overcoming Hurt

DR WINDY DRYDEN

sheldon **PRESS**

First published in Great Britain in 2007

Sheldon Press
36 Causton Street
London SW1P 4ST

British Library Cataloguing-in-Publication Data
A catalogue record for this book is available from the British Library

ISBN: 978–0–85969–914–3

1 3 5 7 9 10 8 6 4 2

Typeset by Fakenham Photosetting Ltd, Fakenham, Norfolk
Printed and bound in Great Britain by Ashford Colour Press

Contents

Part 1

UNDERSTAND HURT AND ITS HEALTHY ALTERNATIVE, SORROW

In this first part of the book, I will begin by introducing you to the basic ideas behind Rational Emotive Behaviour Therapy, the therapeutic approach on which this book is based. Then, I will help you to understand hurt and its healthy alternative, sorrow, from an REBT perspective.

1

Introduction

Like most of my other books for Sheldon Press, this book is based on the therapy approach known as Rational Emotive Behaviour Therapy (REBT). This approach was founded in 1955 by Dr Albert Ellis, an American clinical psychologist who is currently regarded as the grandfather of cognitive behaviour therapy (CBT), the most frequently recommended approach for the treatment of psychological disorders by the National Institute of Clinical Excellence (NICE).

What I am going to do is to outline REBT's Situational ABCDE model in a general way so that you can have some idea of the approach to hurt that I am going to take in this book. If this approach makes sense to you, then I hope you will use the rest of the book in a *practical* way, as this is the best way to get the most out of REBT.

The Situational ABCDE model of REBT

The Situational ABCDE model has six components:

- Situation;
- 'A';
- 'B';
- 'C';
- 'D';
- 'E'.

Let's look at each of these.

Situation

You do not experience an emotional problem in a vacuum. Rather, there is almost always a situation in which you experience this problem. In considering this situation, bear in mind that it should reflect as accurately as possible the context in which you experienced your emotional problem.

'A'

When you experience an emotional problem in the situation that you are in, you usually disturb yourself about a particular aspect of this situation. In REBT, we call this the 'A', or adversity.

'A' is often an inference

It is important to appreciate that your 'A' is usually an inference that you have made about the situation or some aspect of the situation. An inference goes beyond the data at hand and can be accurate or inaccurate. Thus, if you receive a note from your boss saying that he wants to see you after lunch and you think: 'He is going to criticize my work,' then this thought is an inference since it goes beyond the facts of the situation. In this example, the facts are that your boss wants to see you after lunch. You do not know why. Your inference may be accurate or it may be inaccurate, but what makes it an inference is that it goes beyond the data at hand.

'A' relates to your personal domain

An adversity (real or perceived) is usually related to some aspect of your personal domain. The term 'personal domain' was first introduced by Aaron Temkin Beck, the founder of cognitive therapy (an approach to cognitive behaviour therapy which shares certain ideas with REBT). Your personal domain is made up of people, objects, concepts and ideas that are important to you. It also contains what is important to you about yourself. When you experience different unhealthy negative emotions, you disturb yourself about different adversities within your personal domain.

'B'

'B' stands for beliefs. In REBT beliefs can be irrational or rational.

Irrational beliefs and psychological disturbance

REBT's position on psychological disturbance can be summed up as follows:

> People are disturbed not by adversities, but by their rigid and extreme views of adversities.

In REBT, these rigid and extreme views are known as irrational beliefs, and as such are placed under 'B' in the Situational ABCDE model. For example, threats to your personal domain at 'A' do not make you anxious. Rather, you make yourself anxious by holding irrational beliefs at 'B' about such threats.

Apart from being rigid and extreme, irrational beliefs are inconsistent with reality; they are illogical or nonsensical; and they are largely unconstructive in their consequences.

Rational beliefs and psychological health

REBT's position on psychological health can also be summed up thus:

> People respond healthily to adversities by holding flexible and non-extreme views of these adversities.

In REBT, these flexible and non-extreme views are known as rational beliefs and they are also placed under 'B' in the Situational ABCDE model. Thus, you are concerned, but not anxious about threats to your personal domain at 'A' because you hold rational beliefs about such threats at 'B'.

Apart from being flexible and non-extreme, rational beliefs are consistent with reality; they are logical or sensible; and they are largely constructive in their consequences.

REBT theory posits four irrational beliefs and their rational alternatives. These are summarized in Table 1, but I will discuss them in more detail later in this book.

'C'

When you hold a set of beliefs about an adversity, REBT recognizes that there are major consequences (at 'C') of holding these beliefs.

Irrational belief	Rational belief
Demand	Non-dogmatic preference
X must (or must not happen).	I would like x to happen (or not happen), but it does not have to be the way I want it to be.
Awfulizing belief	Anti-awfulizing belief
It would be terrible if x happens (or does not happen).	It would be bad, but not terrible, if x happens (or does not happen).
LFT belief	HFT belief
I could not bear it if x happens (or does not happen).	It would be difficult to bear if x happens (or does not happen), but I could bear it and it would be worth it to me to do so.
Depreciation belief	Acceptance belief
If x happens (or does not happen), I am no good/you are no good/ life is no good.	If x happens (or does not happen), it does not prove that I am no good/ you are no good/life is no good. Rather, I am a FHB/you are a FHB/ life is a complex mixture of good, bad and neutral.

FHB = Fallible human being
LFT = Low frustration tolerance
HFT = High frustration tolerance

Table 1   Irrational and rational beliefs in REBT theory

Three major consequences of beliefs

In REBT, we particularly look for three major consequences of beliefs at 'B':

- emotional;
- behavioural;
- thinking.

Consequences of holding irrational beliefs

The influence of holding irrational beliefs on your emotions, behaviours and subsequent thinking can be summed up as follows:

When you face an adversity and your set of beliefs is irrational, the consequences of these beliefs are likely to be as follows:
'C' (emotional) = largely negative and unhealthy;
'C' (behavioural = largely dysfunctional;
'C' (thinking) = largely negatively distorted and skewed.

In this book I will deal with all three consequences of hurt-based irrational beliefs.

Consequences of holding rational beliefs

The influence of holding rational beliefs on your emotions, behaviours and subsequent thinking can be summed up as follows:

When you face an adversity and your set of beliefs is rational, the consequences of these beliefs are likely to be as follows:
'C' (emotional) = largely negative and healthy;
'C' (behavioural) = largely functional;
'C' (thinking) = largely realistic and balanced.

'D'

In REBT theory, 'D' stands for disputing beliefs, although as you will see I prefer the term 'questioning' to the term 'disputing'. As I discuss questioning (or disputing) beliefs fully in Chapter 3, I will not go into further detail here.

'E'

'E' stands for the effects of disputing or questioning beliefs. When this process is successful, you will experience healthy (rather than unhealthy) negative emotions about life's adversities, functional behavioural responses to these adversities and realistic and balanced ways of thinking about these adversities and their consequences. These healthy ways of thinking, feeling and behaving will help you to change life's adversities if they can be changed, or to adjust constructively to them if they cannot be changed.

If REBT's Situational ABCDE model makes sense to you, then hopefully you will benefit from what REBT has to say about hurt and how to deal with it.

2

Understand hurt

In this book, the position that I take is that the feeling we call 'hurt' is an unhealthy negative emotion that you are most likely to feel when people significant to you act in certain ways or when they fail to act in certain ways. As humans, we do not use language to describe our emotions in any universally agreed way. So it is possible that when you say you feel hurt, you are in fact responding healthily. The only way you can tell if your feelings of hurt are unhealthy rather than healthy is to understand the components of (unhealthy) hurt, and this is my aim in this chapter.

The ingredients of hurt feelings

In this section, I will invite you to think of hurt as an emotional experience comprising several ingredients. I will discuss these ingredients one by one and I will begin my discussion by outlining the ingredients of feelings of hurt experienced in specific situations.

Ingredient 1:	Another person acts or fails to act in a certain way. This may refer to one or more people.
Ingredient 2:	You make an inference about their behaviour or lack of behaviour.
Ingredient 3:	You hold a set of beliefs about this inference which is at the core of your experience of hurt. It is the most important ingredient in explaining why you feel hurt as opposed to sorrow, the healthy alternative to hurt. I will consider the ingredients of sorrow in the next chapter.
Ingredient 4:	You subsequently think in ways that are consistent with these beliefs. •
Ingredient 5:	You act in ways that are consistent with these beliefs.

Now let me deal with these issues one at a time.

Ingredient 1: What people do or do not do

You are most likely to feel hurt about what another person has done or has not done. This applies whether it is one person or a number of people who are involved. At this point it is possible to describe with accuracy exactly what it is the other person (in this case) has done. As we shall see later, it is useful to have an objective reference point about what the other person did or did not do. Here are a few examples of the types of behaviour (and non-behaviour) that people point to when they feel hurt:

What people do

- 'My friend, Jill, told another friend, Beryl, something that I told her in confidence.'
- 'I asked Maureen what she thought of my haircut and she said she didn't like it.'
- 'I heard them laughing when they were told I was rejected by my boyfriend.'

What people do not do

- 'My friend, Joan, did not ask me to join her coffee morning group.'
- 'Norman did not reply to my text asking for a favour even though I had done him several favours previously.'
- 'The social group to which I had given my time freely did not thank me for my efforts but thanked Gina for her work, even though she had devoted less time than I did.'

Hurt and other people

We tend to feel hurt about the actions or lack of actions of people who are important to us in some way (sometimes referred to as 'significant others'). Conversely, we are less likely to feel hurt about the treatment we receive at the hands of strangers or those who occupy a more peripheral role in our lives. Feelings of hurt are not caused when others fail to live up to our expectations, but hurt is correlated with these unmet expectations.

Ingredient 2: Hurt-related inferences

In the previous section, I made the point that we tend to feel hurt when other people who are significant to us act or fail to act in certain ways. I suggested that it is useful to describe this behaviour or its absence as objectively as possible because later, when you are ready, you can refer to this description as you test your inferences about this behaviour or its absence against reality.

This point underscores an important fact. When you feel hurt, you make one or more inferences about the ways others act or fail to act. These inferences are, as I have already said, hunches about reality which may be accurate or inaccurate. When you feel hurt, though, you are operating on the basis that these inferences are in fact true.

What follows is a list of common hurt-related inferences about what people have done or failed to do. It is important to note that usually when you feel hurt you consider that you do not deserve such behaviour at the hands of the other person. Indeed, it is very likely that you consider that you deserve the very opposite.

Inferences related to what people have done

In this section, I will concentrate on hurt-related inferences about what people have done.

Being unfairly criticized

While you can feel hurt about unfair or fair criticism, you are more likely to feel hurt about a significant other criticizing you unfairly. In addition, you are more likely to feel hurt about criticism that is directed at you as a person rather than criticism that is directed at your behaviour.

In addition, you tend to feel particularly hurt when someone close to you criticizes you for something that is your Achilles' heel, particularly if you think that this person is doing so knowing that this is a vulnerable area for you.

> Rachel felt hurt whenever her husband criticized her hairstyle, hair and appearance being a vulnerable area for her. She in part based her worth on her appearance. However, these feelings were also related to her inference that her husband criticized her knowing that she was particularly vulnerable to such criticism.

Being rejected

When you feel hurt about being rejected, you focus particularly on the undeserved nature of the rejection. You tend to remind yourself of all the good things that you have done for the person concerned and how you deserve far better treatment from them. You are more likely to feel hurt about rejection when the person who has rejected you is important to you than when they are relatively unimportant.

> Malcolm felt hurt about being rejected by his girlfriend, Sarah. During their relationship, Malcolm had gone out of his way to be kind to her and had helped her when her mother was sick, but she 'dumped' him, as she said, 'when someone with a bit more money came along'.

Being disapproved of

Disapproval is similar to rejection in that they both involve the other person making some kind of negative judgement of you. They are different in that with rejection the other person has cast you aside, something he (in this case) hasn't yet done when he has disapproved of you. As in rejection, when you are disapproved of, you are more likely to feel hurt: (1) when you consider this disapproval to be undeserved rather than deserved; and (2) when the disapproval comes from people who are significant to you rather than from those who are peripheral to you.

> Marie had always prided herself on being a good mother. However, in her therapy group two of the other group members strongly disapproved of her for being overprotective of her children and, as they claimed, for 'discouraging their development'. This coloured their response to anything that she talked about in the group. Marie felt hurt about their disapproval, in particular because she considered it unwarranted.

Being betrayed

Being betrayed by someone you are close to is a key hurt-related inference.

> Fiona placed her trust in Jill, who was a good friend, and told her a secret, making her swear not to tell a living soul. However, a week later Fiona found out that Jill had told their mutual friend, Beryl, the secret. Fiona felt hurt because she considered that Jill had betrayed her trust.

Being used

Being used is another key inference in hurt. When someone uses you, she (in this case) is concealing the true purpose in her dealings with you. She is, in fact, having a relationship solely or mainly for her own selfish ends. I use the term 'selfish' advisedly here, in that such people are rarely concerned about you or your interests. The person who is using you typically does not disabuse you in your assumption that she does care for you and is acting in good faith in her relationship with you. The more the person is important to you, the more you are likely to feel hurt when you discover that you have been used.

> Peter helped Paul when Paul was struggling with his coursework and had fallen behind with his assignments. As soon as Paul had caught up with his work, he did not want to spend much time with Peter, until later when he fell behind with his work again. Then he approached Peter, ostensibly to go out socially, but in reality to seek more help for his work. Peter felt hurt about Paul using him.

Inferences related to what people have failed to do

In this section, I will concentrate on hurt-related inferences about what people have failed to do in their relationship with you. Once again, it is important to note that when you feel hurt it is likely that you consider that you deserve far better treatment than you are getting from the other person.

Being neglected

Inferring that you have been neglected by someone close to you is a common hurt-related inference. Neglect implies that you are not receiving attention that you can reasonably expect from the person in question. A sense of neglect is heightened when others receive the expected attention from the significant other and you do not, as in the example below.

> Marie considered that her mother neglected her at dinner when she asked her sisters about their day at work and didn't ask her. This tended to be a common pattern in the family.

Being unfairly excluded

Being unfairly excluded or left out by a significant other or others when you think you don't deserve to be is another common situation about which people make themselves feel hurt. This often happens in three-person situations, when two people decide to do something and do not include the third person.

Heather felt hurt when her two friends, Joanna and Linda, decided to go to the cinema and did not invite her. She inferred that they had excluded her.

Not being appreciated

Not being appreciated when you think you deserve to be is another situation about which people tend to feel hurt. This is particularly the case when others are appreciated for the same as you have done or even for less. A sense of unfairness often accompanies a sense of being unappreciated.

Marcus felt hurt that his sales record was not appreciated by his MD when the latter showed appreciation for his colleague's slightly inferior sales record.

Being deprived of what you want when you think you have deserved it

As you have now seen, the concept of deservingness is an important one in situations about which you make yourself feel hurt. It is frequently present in situations where you have been deprived of what you want, since when you feel hurt you often think that you do not deserve to be so deprived.

Robert felt hurt when he failed to get a bonus at work which he considered he deserved. He had worked particularly hard for this bonus, often staying behind late to complete tasks that his colleagues left unfinished.

Feelings of hurt about undeserved deprivations tend to be heightened when other people have made promises they don't keep, when the other people concerned are particularly significant and when others less deserving receive what you have been deprived of.

Ingredient 3: Irrational beliefs

This third ingredient is the most important in the experience of hurt. Indeed, I would go as far as to say that without these irrational beliefs, you would not experience hurt even if you made one or more of the inferences listed in the above section. Thus, being unfairly excluded, for example, does not make you feel hurt; rather, you make yourself feel hurt about unfair exclusion by the irrational beliefs that you hold about this actual or inferred event. But what exactly are irrational beliefs?

Four irrational beliefs

As I outlined in Chapter 1, this book is based on an approach to counselling and psychotherapy known as Rational Emotive Behaviour Therapy (REBT), founded over 50 years ago by an American psychologist called Albert Ellis. Dr Ellis's basic idea can be summed up in the following phrase:

> People are disturbed not by things, but by the rigid and extreme beliefs that they hold about things.

Dr Ellis specified what he meant by rigid and extreme beliefs. He argued that rigid beliefs take the form of demands, musts, have to's, oughts, etc. His view is that these rigid beliefs are at the very core of our disturbed feelings like hurt, and that three extreme beliefs are derived from these rigid beliefs, which are also at the root of emotional disturbance. So there are four irrational beliefs:

1 demands;
2 awfulizing beliefs: 'It is awful if my demands are not met';
3 low frustration tolerance (LFT) beliefs: 'I can't bear it when my demands are not met';
4 depreciation beliefs: ' I/you/life is no good when my demands are not met'.

Two types of hurt

Before I discuss the irrational beliefs that are so crucial to the creation and development of hurt feelings, I want to make an important distinction between two types of hurt: ego hurt and non-ego hurt.

Ego hurt

When you make yourself feel hurt in the ego domain, you feel hurt because you are depreciating yourself in some way for the undeserved treatment you have experienced at the hands of a significant other or others.

Non-ego hurt

By contrast, when you make yourself feel hurt in the non-ego domain, you are focusing on how horrible the world is for allowing you be treated in such an unfair way. You are not depreciating yourself for this treatment; rather, you feel sorry for yourself for the way you have been treated.

To complicate matters, it is possible for you to make yourself feel hurt in both ego and non-ego domains about the same event. If this applies to you, it is important that you deal with these different types of hurt one at a time.

Now let me discuss the irrational beliefs that lead to hurt in both these domains. Let me begin with ego hurt.

Irrational beliefs in ego hurt

Ego hurt is underpinned by a rigid belief and an extreme self-depreciation belief. For example:

- a rigid belief (e.g. 'You must not reject me'); and
- a self-depreciation belief (e.g. 'Your rejection makes me unlovable').

Sometimes when unhealthy anger is a feature of hurt you also hold an other-depreciation belief (e.g. 'You are rotten for rejecting me since you are reminding me that I am unlovable').

Irrational beliefs in non-ego hurt

Non-ego hurt is underpinned by a rigid belief and one or more extreme beliefs:

- a rigid demand (e.g. 'You must not betray me');
- an awfulizing belief (e.g. 'It is awful that you betrayed me. Poor me, I don't deserve to be treated like this');
- a low frustration tolerance (LFT) belief (e.g. 'I can't stand being betrayed. Poor me, I don't deserve to be treated like this');
- a life-depreciation belief (e.g. 'Life is rotten for allowing such bad treatment to poor, undeserving me');
- an other-depreciation belief (e.g. 'You are a bad person for betraying poor, undeserving me').This is particularly the case where unhealthy anger is a feature of non-ego hurt.

You will notice that in ego hurt and non-ego hurt there is a different stance towards the self. In ego hurt, your basic stance towards yourself is based on depreciation. Indeed, ego hurt is so called because when you experience it you are depreciating yourself in some way. In non-ego hurt, you are not depreciating yourself; rather you view yourself as hard done by, a poor person who has been harshly and undeservedly treated by life.

To summarize this, we may say that:

- ego hurt is based on self-depreciation;
- non-ego hurt is based on self-pity.

Ingredient 4: Subsequent thinking consistent with your hurt-based irrational beliefs

When you hold a hurt-creating irrational belief about any of the factors I discussed earlier in this chapter (see pp. 11–14), this belief will influence the way that you subsequently think. As you will see, this subsequent thinking is highly distorted. However, if you engage with this subsequent thinking and treat it as accurately reflecting reality rather than as distorted products of your prior irrational beliefs, you will tend to perpetuate your hurt feelings. When you begin to experience hurt, you tend to think in one or more of the following ways:

Exaggerating the unfairness of the other person's behaviour

As I discussed earlier in this chapter, you are much more likely to make yourself feel hurt about being treated badly by those close to you when you consider that you do not deserve such treatment than when you think that you do. When you hold hurt-based irrational beliefs and when you think again about the way you have been treated by the other person, your tendency is to exaggerate how unfairly you have been treated. Specifically, you think about all the good things you have done for the other person and edit out all the good things that he or she has done for you. Consequently, you will dwell on the unfair imbalance that your irrational beliefs encourage you to focus on.

Seeing the other person as showing indifference or a lack of care

When you hold hurt-based irrational beliefs about the unfair treatment that you have experienced at the hands of someone close to you, you then tend to conclude that the reason he (in this case) treated you so badly is that he doesn't care about you or is indifferent towards you. If you think this way, you will focus on his lack of caring or indifference and then disturb yourself about this attitude by thinking irrationally about it, thus deepening your hurt feelings.

Seeing yourself as alone, uncared for or misunderstood

When you hold hurt-based irrational beliefs about being mistreated by a significant other, you then tend to see yourself placed in a negative situation in relation to the world. This view is usually an over-generalization. For example, when someone mistreats you and you make yourself feel hurt about this, you tend to think that you are alone in the world, uncared for in the world or misunderstood by the world. This negative situation will be coloured by ego-based hurt (e.g. 'I am uncared for in the world. This proves that I am not worth caring about') or by non ego-based hurt (e.g. 'I am alone in the world. Poor me!').

Thinking of past 'hurts'

When you have made yourself feel hurt by holding a relevant hurt-based irrational belief, you will tend to focus on other past hurts. Here, you bring to mind all the occasions when you have been mistreated, unappreciated and unfairly rejected by people.

Thinking that the other person has to put things right of his or her own accord

When you have made yourself feel hurt by holding irrational beliefs about what another person has done or not done, you tend to think that this person has to make the first move to put things right between you. You will therefore do nothing to help yourself heal the rift, and as a result your passivity will increase your self-pity and/or self-depreciation, particularly if the other person does not make the first move.

Ingredient 5: Action consistent with your hurt-based irrational beliefs

When you hold a set of irrational beliefs that lead you to feel hurt, you tend to act in certain ways which serve to deepen your experience of hurt. Here is a list of some the main hurt-related behaviours:

Blaming the other person for making you feel hurt

When discussing your feelings of hurt with friends and acquaintances, you tend to place the blame for your hurt feelings on the behaviour of the person with whom you feel hurt, rather than taking responsibility for making yourself feel hurt about what that person did or didn't do.

Shutting down direct channels of communication

When you feel hurt because of your irrational beliefs about what another person has done or not done, you tend to shut down direct channels of communication with the person about whom you have made yourself feel hurt. You are very reluctant to communicate directly with the person and tell him or her what you feel hurt about. However, your goal is to *indirectly* show the other person how you feel. You tend to do this by sulking.

Sulking comes in two major forms. The first involves you not talking to the other person at all. You can either do this loudly (e.g. by banging doors) or quietly (by silently rebuffing all attempts by the other person to engage you in direct communication). The second form of sulking involves you criticizing the other person but not telling that person what you feel hurt about.

As I showed in my book *The Incredible Sulk* (Sheldon Press, 1992), sulking has a number of purposes, all of which are consistent with your goal of making and sustaining your feelings of hurt. The purposes of sulking are as follows:

- Sulking can punish the other person for 'hurting' your feelings.
- Sulking can get what you want from the other person. If your sulking behaviour works, in the sense that you get what you want from the other by sulking, then you are more likely to use it in future.
- Sulking can get the other person to make the first move. Part of the philosophy that underpins hurt is that someone has treated you unfairly and it is up to that person to make efforts to find out how he or she has 'hurt' you. The other person then has to put things right between you. It is also part of this philosophy not to make this process too easy for the other person even if he or she does make the first move.

- Sulking can extract proof of caring from the other person. Here, the other person has to prove that he (in this case) cares for you by making continued attempts to get you to talk. If he doesn't do this or gives up too easily, you have something else to make yourself feel hurt about.
- Sulking can provide protection from further hurt. Here, you stop communicating with the other person because you think that if you continue to communicate with her (in this case), she will keep acting in ways that you will make yourself feel hurt about. To protect yourself, therefore, you stop communicating with her.
- Sulking can restore a sense of power. With this as a motive, your sulking is an attempt to get the upper hand in the relationship with the person who in your mind has hurt you. In doing so you reinforce your hurt-creating irrational beliefs.

When hurt is a general problem for you

In outlining the five ingredients of hurt, I was working on the assumption that you experienced hurt feelings in a specific situation. Now, if you experience hurt feelings in a number of different situations, the following are likely to be the case:

1 It is likely that you hold a general version of the hurt-related irrational beliefs I discussed above.
2 These general irrational beliefs will routinely lead you to make certain types of inferences about the behaviour of others (or their failure to behave in certain ways) along the lines that I discussed earlier in this chapter.
3 Your general hurt-related beliefs will also lead you to act and subsequently think in routine ways that are consistent with these beliefs.

Let me focus on the second of the above principles. This is that you bring your general hurt-related irrational belief to situations where there is some ambiguity, and this belief leads you to make hurt-related inferences in ways that are consistent with the content of your belief.

For example, imagine that you held the following general hurt-based irrational belief (in this case in the non-ego domain): 'Those close to me must include me in everything that they do and it's terrible if they don't. Poor me if I am excluded.'

Imagine bringing this general irrational belief to relevant situations where it is possible that you were not included, although this is not clear. Because you cannot convince yourself that you have not been excluded, you will tend to think that these other people have excluded you, that they have excluded you unfairly and that they did so intentionally. Having created this hurt-based inference, you will then evaluate it using a specific version of this general hurt-based irrational belief and thereby make yourself feel hurt in the specific situation. Your typical thinking and behavioural consequences of these general hurt-related irrational beliefs will follow.

Here is an example of all three principles in action.

> Jim held the following general hurt-based irrational belief: 'Because I would not betray the trust of those close to me, they must not betray my trust, and if they do the world is a rotten place for allowing this to happen to poor, undeserving me.' Jim took this general irrational belief to a specific situation where he learned that his sister, whose confidences he had kept in the past, *may*, when drunk, have told a group of their mutual friends something that he told her in strict confidence. Jim's general hurt-based irrational belief led him to infer that his sister had, in fact, betrayed his trust. It is as if he reasoned: 'Because I can't convince myself that my sister did not betray my trust, then she did. If she did so, she betrayed my trust intentionally.' Jim's belief did not easily allow him to think that his sister had not betrayed his trust or that, if she did, she did so unintentionally because she was drunk. Once Jim created the inference that he was betrayed, he easily made himself feel hurt about it by holding a specific version of his general irrational belief. Thus: 'My sister betrayed my trust intentionally by telling our mutual friends something that I told her in confidence. She absolutely should not have betrayed me and the world is a rotten place for allowing this to happen to poor, undeserving me.'

> Having made himself feel hurt in this way, Jim then thought and acted in ways that were consistent with his feelings of hurt. He thought that his sister had to come to him to apologize profusely for what she had done (even though his sister knew nothing of his feelings), and he sulked for weeks before talking to his sister, but then only about superficial matters.

> Thinking that others had to come to him and sulking were typical thinking and behavioural consequences of Jim's general hurt-related irrational beliefs.

A view of the world from hurt-based irrational beliefs

When your hurt-based irrational beliefs, hurt-related inferences, actions and subsequent types of thinking become entrenched and have become predominant in your life, you can be said to have developed a hurt-based world view.

The world view that renders you vulnerable to feelings of hurt does so primarily because it makes it very easy for you to make hurt-related inferences. You find it easy to make these inferences because of your general hurt-based irrational beliefs. Then, as I have shown you earlier in the chapter, you make yourself feel hurt about these inferences, with the appropriate irrational beliefs. Here is the hurt-based world view and the inferences that it spawns.

> *World view:* When I do a lot for those close to me, they will fail to reciprocate.
> *Inference:* People close to me will let me down.

> *World view:* If I trust those close to me, they will often betray me while I would not betray them.
> *Inference:* People close to me will betray me.

> *World view:* Significant others will treat me unfairly, while I would not be unfair to them.
> *Inference:* I will not get what I deserve from significant others.

> *World view:* Those close to me will often exclude or neglect me for no good reason.
> *Inference:* If I learn that people close to me are doing things together when I have not been invited, this is evidence that I have been excluded or neglected.

In REBT, we argue that, when faced with life's adversities, it is healthy for us to experience healthy negative emotions about these adversities rather than unhealthy negative emotions. In the following chapter, I will therefore discuss 'sorrow', which is the healthy negative emotion alternative to hurt.

3

Understand sorrow: the healthy alternative to feeling hurt

In Rational Emotive Behaviour Therapy (REBT), the approach to therapy on which this book is based, we argue that when we face adversities in life it is healthy to experience a negative emotion. We make a distinction between emotions that are negative in tone and unhealthy in effect (these we call 'unhealthy negative emotions') and emotions that are negative in tone and healthy in effect (which we call 'healthy negative emotions'). In Chapter 2, I explained that 'hurt' is an unhealthy negative emotion and went on to outline the five ingredients that go to make up hurt. In this chapter, I will outline the five ingredients that comprise 'sorrow', which I consider to be the healthy alternative to hurt.

Before I do so, a word about language. I have said that I consider 'sorrow' to be the healthy alternative to hurt. What is important is not the word that I have chosen (i.e. 'sorrow') but the five ingredients that go to make up 'sorrow'. So if it is more meaningful for you to come up with a different term to 'sorrow' as a healthy alternative to hurt, then that's fine. The important thing is that you understand the differences between hurt and whatever you call its healthy alternative.

The ingredients of sorrow

In this section, just as I did with hurt, I will invite you to think of sorrow as an emotional experience comprising five ingredients. As you will see, sorrow is indistinguishable from hurt in the first two of the five ingredients and differs from hurt in the remaining three. As I did in the previous chapter, I will discuss the ingredients of sorrow one by one, and I will begin my discussion by outlining the ingredients of feelings of sorrow experienced in specific situations.

Ingredient 1:	Another person acts or fails to act in a certain way. This may refer to one or more people. This is exactly the same as in hurt.
Ingredient 2:	You make an inference about their behaviour or lack of behaviour. This too is exactly the same as in hurt.
Ingredient 3:	You hold a set of beliefs about this inference which is at the core of your experience of sorrow. It is the most important ingredient in explaining why you feel sorrow as opposed to hurt. As we will see, the beliefs in sorrow are very different from those in hurt.
Ingredient 4:	You subsequently think in ways that are consistent with these beliefs. Your subsequent thinking when you feel sorrow is different from your subsequent thinking in hurt.
Ingredient 5:	You act in ways that are consistent with these beliefs. Again, your behaviour when you feel sorrow is different from your behaviour when you feel hurt.

Now let me deal with these issues one at a time.

Ingredient 1: What people do or do not do

As with hurt, you are most likely to feel sorrow about what another person has done or not done. This again applies whether it is one person or a number of people who are involved. As I stressed in Chapter 2, at this point it is possible to describe with accuracy exactly what it is the other person (in this case) has done. In Chapter 2, I gave a few examples of the types of behaviour (and non-behaviour) that people point to when they feel hurt. These are exactly the same when they feel sorrow, as you will note.

What people do

- 'My friend, Jill, told another friend, Beryl, something that I told her in confidence.'

- 'I asked Maureen what she thought of my haircut and she said she didn't like it.'
- 'I heard them laughing when they were told I was rejected by my boyfriend.'

What people do not do

- 'My friend, Joan, did not ask me to join her coffee morning group.'
- 'Norman did not reply to my text asking for a favour, even though I had done him several favours previously.'
- 'The social group to which I had given my time freely did not thank me for my efforts, but thanked Gina for her work, even though she had devoted less time than I did.'

Sorrow and other people

As with hurt, we tend to feel sorrow about the actions or absence of actions of people who are important to us in some way. Conversely, we are less likely to feel sorrow about the treatment we receive at the hands of strangers or those who occupy a more peripheral role in our lives. As with hurt, feelings of sorrow are not caused when others fail to live up to our expectations, but hurt is correlated with these unmet expectations.

Ingredient 2: Sorrow-related inferences

In specific episodes, the inferences we tend to make about what others have done or have not done when we feel sorrow are exactly the same as when we feel hurt. In the previous section, I made the point that we tend to feel sorrow when other people who are significant to us act or fail to act in certain ways. I suggested that it is useful to describe this behaviour or its absence as objectively as possible because later, when you are ready, you can refer to this description as you test your inferences about this behaviour or its absence against reality.

So when you feel sorrow about the way others have treated you, you make a number of inferences. I will only list them here since they are the same as the inferences you make when you feel hurt. Refer to Chapter 2 for a discussion of these inferences, which are, don't forget, hunches about reality which may be accurate or inaccurate. When you feel sorrow (or hurt), though, you are operating on the basis that these inferences are true.

As with hurt, in sorrow you also consider that you do not deserve such behaviour at the hands of the other person. Indeed, it is very likely that you consider you deserve the very opposite.

Inferences related to what people have done

- You infer you are being unfairly criticized.
- You infer you are being rejected.
- You infer you are being disapproved of.
- You infer you are being betrayed.
- You infer you are being used.

Inferences related to what people have failed to do

- You infer you are being neglected.
- You infer you are being unfairly excluded.
- You infer you are not being appreciated.
- You infer you are being deprived of what you want when you think you have deserved it.

Ingredient 3: Rational beliefs

As with hurt, this third ingredient is the most important in the experience of sorrow. The inferences that you make about others' behaviour, as outlined above, explain why you may feel hurt or sorrow, but they do not explain which of these two emotions you will experience. In the previous chapter, I explained that irrational beliefs are at the core of hurt. Similarly, rational beliefs are at the core of sorrow. But what are rational beliefs?

Four rational beliefs

As I explained in Chapter 1, this book is based on an approach to counselling and psychotherapy known as Rational Emotive Behaviour Therapy (REBT), founded by Dr Albert Ellis. Dr Ellis's basic idea with respect to rational beliefs is that when people hold beliefs that are flexible and non-extreme about life's adversities, they experience healthy negative emotions which reflect the fact that they are facing something negative in their lives and that they are handling it constructively.

Dr Ellis specified what he meant by flexible and non-extreme beliefs. He argued that flexible beliefs take the form of wishes and wants, for example. These beliefs point to our preferences, but make clear, as we will see later, that we do not have to have our preferences met. Ellis's view is that these flexible beliefs are at the very core of our healthy negative feelings like sorrow, and that three non-extreme beliefs are derived from these flexible beliefs. So there are four non-extreme beliefs, which are also at the root of healthy negative feelings:

1 non-dogmatic preferences;
2 anti-awfulizing beliefs: 'It is bad, but not awful, if my preferences are not met';
3 high frustration tolerance (HFT) beliefs: 'It is difficult for me to tolerate it when my preferences are not being met, but I can bear it and it is worth it to me to do so';
4 acceptance beliefs: 'When my preferences are not met and it is due to me, I am not bad, but a fallible human being ... when it is due to you, you are not bad, but a fallible human being ... and when it is due to other circumstances, life is not bad, but a complex mixture of good, bad and neutral.'

Two types of sorrow

Before I discuss the rational beliefs that are so crucial to the creation and development of sorrow, I want to make an important distinction between two types of sorrow: ego sorrow and non-ego sorrow.

Ego sorrow

When you feel sorrow in the ego domain, you are accepting yourself even though you have experienced undeserved treatment at the hands of a significant other or others.

Non-ego sorrow

By contrast, when you feel sorrow in the non-ego domain, you are acknowledging that it is bad, but not horrible, that you have been treated in such an unfair way. You do not feel sorry for yourself for being in this poor situation.

Now let me discuss the rational beliefs that lead to sorrow in both of these domains. Let me begin with ego sorrow.

Rational beliefs in ego sorrow

Ego sorrow is underpinned by a non-dogmatic preference and a non-extreme self-acceptance belief. For example:

- a non-dogmatic preference belief (e.g. 'I don't want you to reject me, but it does not mean that you must not do so'); and
- a self-acceptance belief (e.g. 'Your rejection does not change me. I am the same fallible human being whether you reject me or not').

Rational beliefs in non-ego sorrow

Non-ego sorrow is underpinned by a flexible belief and one or more non-extreme beliefs:

- a non-dogmatic preference (e.g. 'I don't want you to betray me, but that does not mean that you must not do so');
- an anti-awfulizing belief (e.g. 'It is bad, but not awful, that you betrayed me. While I don't deserve to be treated like this, this is a poor situation, but I am not a poor person');
- a high frustration tolerance (HFT) belief (e.g. 'It is difficult for me to put up with being betrayed, but I can stand it and it is worth it to me to do so ... While I don't deserve to be treated like this, this is a poor situation, but I am not a poor person');
- a life-acceptance belief (e.g. 'Life is not rotten for allowing such bad treatment to happen to me. It is a complex mixture of good, bad and neutral and I am not a poor person for receiving such poor treatment');
- an other-acceptance (e.g. 'You are not a bad person for betraying me. You are a fallible human being who acted badly').

Ingredient 4: Subsequent thinking consistent with your sorrow-based rational beliefs

When you hold a sorrow-creating rational belief about any of the factors I discussed earlier in this chapter (see pp. 25–6), this belief will influence the way that you subsequently think. The subsequent thinking you engage in when you feel sorrow is realistic. Thus, when you begin to experience sorrow, you tend to think in one or more of the following ways:

Viewing the unfairness of the other person's behaviour

When you hold sorrow-related rational beliefs about being treated unfairly by another person and you reflect on this situation, you are more likely to think realistically about the other person's behaviour than if you were holding hurt-related irrational beliefs. Thus, you will tend to view the unfairness of the other person in context and without due exaggeration.

As I discussed earlier in this chapter, you are much more likely to make yourself feel sorrow about being treated badly by those close to you. While you may well think about all the good things you have done for the other person, you will also think about all the good things they have done for you.

Seeing the other person as having complex motives

When you hold sorrow-based rational beliefs about the unfair treatment that you have experienced at the hands of someone close to you, you then tend to conclude that the reason she (in this case) treated you so badly is complex rather than rushing to the conclusion, as you do when you are thinking irrationally (and feeling hurt), that she doesn't care about you or is indifferent towards you. You will still think she cares for you, but at that moment her behaviour is guided by other, perhaps more self-oriented considerations.

Seeing yourself as in a poor situation

When you hold sorrow-based rational beliefs about being mistreated by a significant other, you then tend to see yourself placed in a negative situation, but not in relation to the world as you do when you feel hurt. This view is therefore a realistic one. For example, when someone mistreats you and you make yourself feel sorrow but not hurt about this, you think that you have been treated badly, but you do not think that you are alone in the world, uncared for in the world or misunderstood by the world.

Thinking in a balanced way about past treatment from people

When you have made yourself feel sorrow by holding a relevant rational belief, you will tend to think about past treatment from people in a balanced way. Thus, you will recognize that you have been treated both well and badly in the past, rather than focusing on all the occasions you have been mistreated, unappreciated and unfairly rejected by people, which is what you do when you feel hurt.

Thinking about how to raise the issue with the other person

When you have made yourself feel sorrow by holding rational beliefs about what another person has done or not done, you tend to think about how best to raise the issue with the other person so he or she puts things right, rather than thinking that this person has to make the first move to put things right between you. You will therefore think about how best to heal the rift and think proactively, rather than passively as you do when you feel hurt.

Ingredient 5: Action consistent with your sorrow-based rational beliefs

When you hold a set of rational beliefs which lead you to feel sorrow, you tend to act in certain ways. Here is a list of some the main sorrow-related behaviours:

Accepting the other person who treated you badly

When, with friends and acquaintances, you are discussing your feelings of sorrow about the way that the other person has treated you, you accept responsibility for your feelings of sorrow. You recognize that the other person has treated you badly, hold him (in this case) responsible for his behaviour, but do not blame him for his actions towards you.

Maintaining direct channels of communication with the other person who has treated you badly

When you feel sorrow because of your rational beliefs about what another person has done or not done, you tend to maintain direct channels of communication with the person about whom you feel sorrow, rather than shutting these channels down, which is what you do when you feel hurt. You communicate directly with the person and tell him or her what you feel sorrowful about rather than sulk, as you do when you feel hurt. It is this direct communication that gives you a sense of power.

When you feel much sorrow in your life

In outlining the five ingredients of sorrow, I was working on the assumption that you experienced feelings of sorrow in a specific situation. Now, if you experience sorrowful feelings in a number of different situations, the following are likely to be the case:

- As I discussed in Chapter 2, when you hold general hurt-related irrational beliefs, you bring these beliefs to situations and infer that people are treating you badly when there is no clear-cut evidence that this is the case. However, when you feel a lot of sorrow in your life (rather than hurt), then there is clear-cut evidence that people are treating you badly and your inferences are, in fact, accurate.
- You hold a general version of the sorrow-related rational beliefs I discussed above and use specific versions of these beliefs to evaluate how you are being treated in specific situations.
- Your general and specific sorrow-related beliefs lead you to act and subsequently think in routine ways that are consistent with these beliefs.

When you feel much sorrow in your life because many people are treating you badly, you are responding healthily to these events. However, because so many people are treating you badly, it is likely that you may have problems in other areas of your life which need attention.

Let me outline two possibilities for your consideration and recommend some self-help reading if you recognize your problem in one of the following descriptions:

1 You are putting up with bad behaviour from others without protest. As a result, you get more of such behaviour from some people. If this is the case, your problem is lack of self-assertion and I suggest that you consult a book I wrote with my colleague Daniel Constantinou, entitled *Assertiveness Step by Step* (Sheldon Press, 2004).

2 You have an anger problem and are reacting angrily to people. They, in turn, act angrily towards you, which you consider to be unfair. Your unhealthy anger is affecting you in two ways, therefore. First, you are reaping what you sow with other people. The reciprocity effect in human behaviour states that others tend to treat you in ways in which you treat them. Thus, others are responding angrily to your displays of anger towards them. Second, if you think that others are treating you unfairly in their response to your unhealthy anger, you are failing to see the effect of your behaviour and think, somewhat narcissistically, that you are right and others are wrong. If unhealthy anger is your problem, consult my book *Overcoming Anger: When Anger Helps and When It Hurts* (Sheldon Press, 1996).

A view of the world from sorrow-based rational beliefs

In Chapter 2, I discussed the world view that renders you vulnerable to feelings of hurt. I argued there that this view has its power primarily because it makes it very easy for you to make hurt-related inferences. When you hold general sorrow-related rational beliefs, then you will tend only to make hurt-related inferences when there is clear-cut evidence for you to do so. This leads to a world view that is more balanced than in hurt. In Table 2, I list the hurt-related world view and typical inferences in the left-hand column, with the corresponding sorrow-related world view and typical inferences in the right-hand column.

Hurt-related	Sorrow-related
World view: When I do a lot for those close to me, they will fail to reciprocate. *Inference:* People close to me will let me down.	*World view:* When I do a lot for people, most will reciprocate, but some will not. *Inference:* Only a few people close to me will let me down.
World view: If I trust those close to me, they will often betray me while I would not betray them. *Inference:* People close to me will betray me.	*World view:* I will not betray the trust of those close to me and they will usually not betray me, although a minority will. *Inference:* Only a few people close to me will betray me.
World view: Significant others will treat me unfairly, while I would not be unfair to them. *Inference:* I will not get what I deserve from significant others.	*World view:* I will be fair to significant others and they will in the main be fair to me, although a few won't. *Inference:* I will get what I deserve from most significant others, but not all.
World view: Those close to me will often exclude or neglect me for no good reason. *Inference:* If I learn that people close to me are doing things together when I have not been invited, this is evidence that I have been excluded or neglected.	*World view:* Those close to me may exclude me or neglect me for no good reason, but will only do so rarely. *Inference:* If I learn that people close to me are doing things together when I have not been invited, then there is probably a good reason why I was not invited.

Table 2 Hurt-related and sorrow-related world views and inferences

In the next chapter, I discuss how to deal with specific episodes of hurt.

Part 2

DEAL WITH SPECIFIC EPISODES OF HURT

So far in this book, I have explained why you feel hurt and discussed the five ingredients that comprise your hurt experience. I then considered sorrow, which I argued is the healthy alternative to hurt, and discussed the five ingredients that comprise sorrow.

In this part of the book, I will show you how to deal with specific episodes of hurt. More specifically, I will outline steps that you need to take in dealing with any specific hurt episode.

4

Define your target problem and be goal-oriented

In any change-related endeavour, you need to define your problem and be clear about what you want to achieve.

Choose one problem to work on

You may have several problems, but in this book I will focus on your hurt feelings. The therapy on which this book is based, Rational Emotive Behaviour Therapy (REBT), works best when you focus on one problem at a time. Your chosen problem, hurt, is known in REBT as a target problem – stick with it as you go through the steps outlined in this part of the book.

To illustrate the points I make in this part of the book, I will use the example of Fiona, whom we met briefly in Chapter 2 (see p. 12).

Describe your target problem

State your target problem as clearly as you can. A good description contains your disturbed feelings (at 'C' in the ABCDE framework outlined in Chapter 1) and what adversity (at 'A') you feel disturbed about.

Fiona's example
'I feel hurt ("C") whenever I consider that I have been betrayed by those close to me ("A").'

Assess for the presence of a meta-emotional problem

Having made yourself hurt in the first place, being human you may disturb yourself about your original disturbance. In REBT this is known as a meta-emotional problem (literally, an emotional problem about an emotional problem or a behavioural problem).

Ask yourself: 'How do I feel about feeling hurt?'

Common meta-emotional problems about hurt are shame, guilt and anger about self. If you do have a meta-emotional problem, you need to decide which of your two problems – the original feelings of hurt or the meta-emotional problem – will be your target problem, the one that will become the focus of your self-help.

My advice is that you should focus on your original target problem of hurt, unless:

- you want to work on your meta-emotional problem first;
- the existence of your meta-emotional problem will interfere with you working on your original target problem of hurt in your life.

If you choose to work on your meta-emotional problem first, then you may need to consult one of my other books before reading this one (e.g. *Overcoming Guilt*, 1994; *Overcoming Shame*, 1997; *Overcoming Anger*, 1996; all Sheldon Press).

Establish a goal orientation

If you have described your hurt problem in general terms, you need to establish a goal orientation. In doing so, understand that you need to react healthily to the adversity at 'A' before trying to change it directly. Setting a general goal direction is acceptable at this point. You will set specific goals later.

Ask yourself: 'What would I like to achieve from focusing on this hurt problem?'

If you want to change a situation or another person, realize that this is not an acceptable goal in REBT. This is because neither situations nor other people are under your direct control. However, you can change your own behaviour, which may have a positive impact on the situation or on others. If you take this route, realize that you need to be in a healthy frame of mind to do this effectively, and this is best achieved by first dealing with your hurt feelings about the situation or about others.

Fiona's example
Fiona recognized that her feelings of hurt were a problem for her. She wanted to handle betrayal more appropriately and without feeling such emotional pain.

5

Assess a concrete example of your hurt

Select a concrete example of your hurt

Once you have defined your hurt problem, select a concrete example of this problem. Working with a concrete example will help you to identify a specific 'A' and a specific 'C' which will later help you to identify a specific irrational belief ('iB'). A concrete example is one that occurred in a specific situation at a specific time with a specific person or persons.

If you find it difficult to select a concrete example of your target problem, pick an example which is fresh in your mind. This example might be:

- recent;
- vivid; or
- typical.

Describe the situation as objectively as you can

Once you have chosen the concrete example of your hurt, describe the situation where you felt hurt as specifically and objectively as you can. Such a description contains no interpretations of what happened and as such is what can be seen and heard on an audio-visual record of the situation.

Fiona's example
Here is Fiona's description of the situation in her selected example: 'I told Jill that I had met a man and asked her not to tell anyone. She told Beryl about it.'

Identify 'C'

In this section, identify your major feeling at 'C', how you acted (or felt like acting) when you experienced hurt and how you subsequently thought.

Emotional 'C'

While your 'C' should be hurt, it may be that you experienced other feelings in the specific example you have selected, e.g. unhealthy anger. Since this is a book on hurt, concentrate on your feelings of hurt.

Behavioural 'C'

Ask yourself: 'When you felt hurt in the episode under consideration what did you feel like doing, but didn't do?'

These behaviours are known as action tendencies. Also identify any behaviours that were designed to help you stop feeling hurt or minimize these feelings.

Thinking 'C'

When you feel hurt, you then tend to have thoughts that are highly distorted and/or designed to help you manage or limit your hurt experience.

Fiona's example
- Emotional 'C' = Hurt.
- Behavioural 'C' = Avoiding Jill, and
  = 'Telling my friends that I felt hurt about Jill's behaviour and stating to them that it was terrible that she acted in that way, agreeing with their irrationalities about the way I was treated.'
- Thinking 'C' = Thinking of ways of avoiding Jill, and the following thoughts:
  = 'All my friends betray me in the end',
  'Everyone will find out about my secret',
  'I will become a laughing stock.'

I will consider behavioural 'Cs' in Chapter 11 in greater detail, and thinking 'Cs' in Chapters 11 and 12.

Identify 'A'

You will recall from Chapter 1 that I made a distinction between 'A' (the adversity in the situation about which you were most disturbed) and the situation in which you were disturbed. 'A' is usually an inference, while the situation is descriptive.

When you assess the 'A' in your selected example, consider two questions:

Ask yourself: 'What was I most hurt by when … (state the situation)?'

Fiona's example
'What was I most hurt by when Jill told Beryl what I asked her to keep to herself?'
Answer: 'That Jill betrayed my trust.'

Ask yourself: 'What one thing would have eliminated or significantly reduced my feelings of hurt when … (state the situation)?' The opposite is your 'A'.

Fiona's example
'What one thing would have eliminated or significantly reduced my feelings of hurt when Jill told Beryl what I asked her to keep to herself?'
Answer: 'Knowing that Jill had not betrayed my trust.'

Common hurt-related inferences

In identifying your hurt-related inferences you might find the following list of common hurt-related inferences useful. I discussed these more fully in Chapter 2.

Inferences related to what people have done

- You infer you are being unfairly criticized.
- You infer you are being rejected.
- You infer you are being disapproved of.

- You infer you are being betrayed.
- You infer you are being used.

Inferences related to what people have failed to do

- You infer you are being neglected.
- You infer you are being unfairly excluded.
- You infer you are not being appreciated.
- You infer you are being deprived of what you want when you think you have deserved it.

Once you have identified your 'A', it is very important that you resist any temptation to challenge 'A', even if it is obviously distorted. Assume temporarily that your 'A' is true. This will enable you to identify your irrational beliefs later.

This is so important, let me repeat it:

> Assume temporarily that your 'A' is true.

You will have an opportunity to re-examine your 'A' later.

Understand the 'B–C' connection

At this point you need to understand that your hurt feelings at 'C' are not determined by the situation or by your inference at 'A', but largely by your beliefs at 'B'. This is known as the 'B–C' connection. So:

> Ask yourself: 'Were my feelings of hurt determined by ... (state "A") or by my beliefs ("B") about ... (state "A")?'

Fiona's example
'Were my feelings of hurt determined by me being betrayed by Jill or by my beliefs about her betrayal?'

If Fiona's answer shows that she understands the 'B–C' connection then she can proceed to the next step. If not, she can use the following method, known as the 100-person technique: 'Would 100 people of my age and gender all feel hurt about ... (state "A")?'

Fiona's example
Would 100 women aged 38 all feel hurt about their friend betraying their trust? If Fiona says no, then she can probably see that the reason 100 people have different feelings about 'A' is that they have different beliefs about 'A'. She can see the 'B–C' connection.

If after this you still cannot see the 'B–C' connection, you might find it helpful to review Chapters 1, 2 and 3 and/or read the first six steps of my book, *Ten Steps to Positive Living* (Sheldon Press, 1994).

Identify your irrational beliefs and see their rational belief alternatives

You have seen that your beliefs underpin your feelings. You are now ready to identify the irrational beliefs (at 'B') that underpinned your feelings of hurt at 'C'. As we saw in Chapter 2, there are four irrational beliefs:

> *Demand:* X must (or must not) happen.
> *Awfulizing belief:* It would be terrible if x happens (or does not happen).
> *LFT belief:* I could not bear it if x happens (or does not happen).
> *Depreciation belief:* If x happens (or does not happen), I am no good/you are no good/life is no good.

And there are four alternative rational beliefs:

> *Non-dogmatic preference:* I would like x to happen (or not happen), but it does not have to be the way I want it to be.
> *Anti-awfulizing belief:* It would be bad, but not terrible, if x happens (or does not happen).
> *HFT belief:* It would be difficult to bear if x happens (or does not happen), but I could bear it and it would be worth it to me to do so.
> *Acceptance belief:* If x happens (or does not happen), it does not prove that I am no good/you are no good/life is no good. Rather, I am a fallible human being/you are a fallible human being/life is a complex mixture of good, bad and neutral.

Your minimum goal at this point is to identify your demand and the one other irrational belief that accounted for your hurt feelings in the situation under consideration.

How can you best do this? By using the following strategy.

Decide what underpinned your hurt feelings

First, take the demand and the non-dogmatic preference and select which underpinned your hurt feelings. 'When I was feeling hurt about ... (state "A"), was I demanding that ... or was I wanting but not demanding that ... (state "A")?'

Fiona's example
'When I was feeling hurt about being betrayed by Jill, was I demanding that she must not betray me or was I wanting her not to betray me, but not demanding that she must not do so?' I was demanding that she must not betray me.

If you cannot see that your demand underpinned your hurt feelings, review Chapters 2 and 3.

Identify your irrational belief*

Once you have identified your demand, select the one other irrational belief (awfulizing belief, LFT belief or depreciation belief) that best accounted for your hurt feelings at 'C'. If your hurt was an example of ego hurt, select your demand and your self-depreciation belief. However, if your hurt was an example of non-ego hurt, select your demand and either your anti-awfulizing belief, LFT belief or life-depreciation belief. You now have identified your demand plus one other irrational belief.

Identify your preference and rational belief*

Now identify your non-dogmatic preference plus one other rational belief. These will help you to achieve your goals.

Fiona's example
'My non-dogmatic preference is "I would really have preferred it if Jill had not betrayed me, but unfortunately she doesn't have to do what I want her to do"'.

---

* When using Fiona's example in the chapters that follow, I will identify and show you how she questioned *all* of her irrational beliefs and rational alternative beliefs.

6

Prepare yourself for the belief-questioning process

Understand the 'iB–C' and 'rB–new C' connections

You have identified your irrational beliefs and alternative rational beliefs. You now need to understand two connections:

1 You need to understand the connection between your irrational beliefs and your feelings of hurt at 'C', known as the *'iB–C' connection*. You have already done this in Chapter 5, but review it if necessary.

2 You also need to understand the connection between your rational beliefs and the alternative healthy negative emotion to hurt – which, as discussed in Chapter 3, is sorrow – known as the *'rB–new C' connection*. This is how you can make this connection. Ask yourself: 'Can I see that as long as I believe ... (state "iBs"), then I will feel hurt? On the other hand, can I see that if I believe ... (state "rBs"), then I will feel sorrow?'

Fiona's example

'Can I see that as long as I believe that Jill absolutely should not have betrayed my trust, then I will feel hurt? On the other hand, can I see that if I believe that it would have been better if she had not betrayed my trust but, sadly and regretfully, this does not mean that she absolutely should not have done so, then I will feel sorrow?'

You need to understand these two connections before engaging in the belief-questioning process to be described in the chapters that follow. If you are having difficulty doing so, again review the material in Chapters 1, 2 and 3.

Commit to pursue feeling sorrow rather than hurt

> Make a commitment to pursue feeling sorrow rather than hurt and understand that changing your irrational beliefs is the best way of doing this.

I discussed above that you need to see that sorrow constitutes the healthy alternative to your hurt feelings at 'C'. After you have done this, you need to make a commitment to work towards this healthy emotion before attempting to change 'A' or the situation.

If you want to change 'A' or the situation, understand that the best time to do this is when you are not disturbed about 'A' or the situation (in this case, when you feel sorrow and not hurt) and that your hurt feelings will interfere with your change attempts. Once you have understood this and know that the best way to be undisturbed about 'A' is by thinking rationally about it, you are ready to question your irrational beliefs about 'A'.

Why question your beliefs?

> The purpose of questioning your beliefs is for you to see that your irrational beliefs are irrational and that your rational beliefs are rational.

When you question your beliefs (both irrational and rational) your goal is to help yourself see that your irrational beliefs are irrational and your rational beliefs are rational. Strengthening your conviction in your rational belief and weakening your conviction in your irrational belief comes later.

Table 3 shows the characteristics of both sets of belief, and you should employ these characteristics in your questioning.

Irrational belief	Rational belief
Rigid or extreme	Flexible or non-extreme
False	True
Illogical	Logical
Leads to unconstructive results	Leads to constructive results

Table 3 Characteristics of irrational beliefs and rational beliefs

Question both irrational and rational beliefs

As I said above, the purpose of questioning beliefs is to encourage you to see that your irrational beliefs are irrational and your rational beliefs are rational. This is known as *intellectual insight*, because while you may understand this point you may not yet have deep conviction in it, to the extent that it influences for the better your feelings and behaviour. This *emotional insight* will come about later, and in Chapter 11 I will teach you some techniques to help you in this respect.

To achieve such intellectual insight, you have to question both your irrational beliefs and your rational beliefs.

Please note that I suggest you question your demand and non-dogmatic preference and, at least, the one other irrational belief and rational belief that you can see is the most appropriate derivative.

I recommend that you question one irrational belief and one rational belief at a time, but always question them together:

Question the demand and the alternative non-dogmatic preference.
Question the awfulizing belief and the alternative anti-awfulizing belief.
Question the LFT belief and the alternative HFT belief.
Question the depreciation belief and the alternative acceptance belief.

In the next four chapters I will illustrate these points, continuing to use the example of Fiona, who felt hurt about her friend Jill betraying her trust when she told Beryl her secret. Although in reality Fiona felt non-ego hurt, I will also use her example in the questioning self-depreciation and self-acceptance beliefs section, for continuity.

7

Question your demand and your non-dogmatic preference

I recommend that you use three main questions when questioning your demand and non-dogmatic preference: the empirical question, the logical question and the pragmatic question. Then you can ask which belief you want to strengthen and which you want to weaken, and why.

First, focus on your demand and your non-dogmatic preference alternative. Write these down side by side, like this:

Demand	Non-dogmatic preference
X must (or must not) happen.	I would like x to happen (or not happen), but it does not have to be the way I want it to be.

Then move on to the three questions. I will present them in a certain order but this is only a guide – other orders are fine.

The empirical question

Ask yourself: 'Which of the following beliefs is true and which is false, and why?'

iB: My demand..

....

rB: My non-dogmatic preference..

....

According to REBT theory, the only correct answer to this question is that the non-dogmatic preference is true and the demand is false. Note the following:

- A rigid demand is inconsistent with reality. For such a demand to be true, the demanded conditions would already have to exist when they do not. Or as soon as you make your demand then these demanded conditions would have to come into existence. Both positions are patently inconsistent with reality.
- On the other hand, a non-dogmatic preference is true, since its two component parts are true. You can prove that you have a particular desire and can provide reasons why you want what you want. You can also prove that you do not have to get what you desire.

Fiona's example

Question: 'Which of the following beliefs is true and which is false, and why?'

- *Demand:* 'Jill absolutely should not have betrayed my trust by telling Beryl my secret.'
- *Non-dogmatic preference:* 'I would really have preferred it if Jill had not betrayed my trust by telling Beryl my secret, *but* unfortunately she doesn't have to do what I want her to do.'

Answer: 'My non-dogmatic preference is true and my demand is false.'

- My rigid demand – that Jill absolutely should not have betrayed me by telling Beryl my secret – is inconsistent with reality. The reality is that she did betray my trust and my demand is my attempt to make reality the way I want it to be. Sadly, I don't have such control! For if I did, my demand would have prevented Jill from telling Beryl my secret.
- On the other hand, my non-dogmatic preference – that I would really have preferred it if Jill had not betrayed my trust by telling Beryl my secret *but* unfortunately she doesn't have to do what I want her to do – is true. It is certainly true that I would have preferred it if Jill had not betrayed my trust and it is also true that she didn't have to do what I would have preferred.

The logical question

Ask yourself: 'Which of the following beliefs is logical and which is illogical, and why?'

iB: My demand...

....

rB: My non-dogmatic preference..

....

According to REBT theory your demand is illogical, while your non-dogmatic preference is logical. Your demand is based on the same desire as your non-dogmatic preference, but you transform it as follows:

I prefer that x happens (or does not happen) ... and therefore this absolutely must (or must not) happen.

This belief has two components. The first – 'I prefer that x happens (or does not happen)' – is not rigid, but the second – 'and therefore this must (or must not) happen' – is rigid. As such your rigid demand is not logical, since one cannot logically derive something rigid from something that is not rigid. The template in Figure 1 illustrates this.

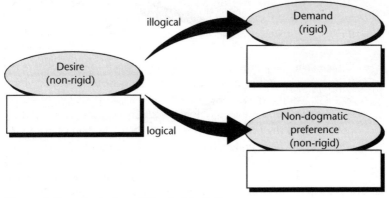

Figure 1 Your logical and illogical beliefs

Your non-dogmatic preference is as follows:

> I prefer that *x* happens (or does not happen) ... but this does not mean that it must (or must not) happen.

Your non-dogmatic preference is logical, since both parts are not rigid, and thus the second component logically follows from the first. Again, the template in Figure 1 illustrates this.

Fiona's example
Question: 'Which of the following beliefs is logical and which is illogical, and why?'

- *Demand:* 'Jill absolutely should not have betrayed my trust by telling Beryl my secret.'
- *Non-dogmatic preference:* 'I would really have preferred it if Jill had not betrayed my trust by telling Beryl my secret, *but* unfortunately she doesn't have to do what I want her to do.'

Answer: 'My non-dogmatic preference is logical and my demand is illogical.'

- My rigid demand – that Jill absolutely should not have betrayed me by telling Beryl my secret – is illogical. This rigid belief has two components. The first component is based on my preference 'I wish Jill had not betrayed my trust in this way' and is not rigid. The second component 'and therefore she absolutely should not have done so' is rigid. Therefore my demand is illogical, since one cannot logically derive something rigid from something that is not rigid. This is illustrated in Figure 2.

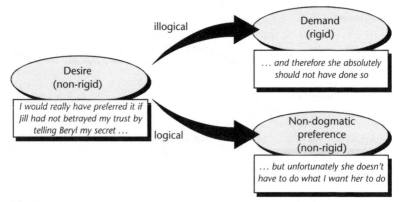

Figure 2 Why Fiona's demand is illogical and her non-dogmatic preference is logical

- On the other hand, my non-dogmatic preference is logical. This rigid belief also has two components. The first component is based on my preference 'I wish Jill had not betrayed my trust in this way' and is not rigid. The second component *'but* unfortunately she does not have to do what I want her to do' is also not rigid. Therefore my non-dogmatic preference is logical, since its two components are not rigid and are therefore logically connected together, as also shown in Figure 2.

The pragmatic question

Ask yourself: 'Which of the following beliefs leads to largely healthy results and which leads to largely unhealthy results and why?'

iB: My demand...

....

rB: My non-dogmatic preference...

....

You need to acknowledge that your demand leads to unhealthy results for you, while your non-dogmatic preference leads to healthier results. Write down the consequences of holding both beliefs and refer, if necessary, to the section headed 'Understand the "iB–C" and "rB–new C" connections' on p. 46.

Fiona's example
Question: 'Which of the following beliefs leads to largely healthy results and which leads to largely unhealthy results, and why?'
- *Demand:* 'Jill absolutely should not have betrayed my trust by telling Beryl my secret.'
- *Non-dogmatic preference:* 'I would really have preferred it if Jill had not betrayed my trust by telling Beryl my secret, *but* unfortunately she doesn't have to do what I want her to do.'

Answer: 'My non-dogmatic preference leads to healthy results, while my rigid demand leads to unhealthy results.'
- When I believe 'I would really have preferred it if Jill had not betrayed my trust by telling Beryl my secret, *but* unfortunately she doesn't have to do what I want her to do', I feel sorrowful rather than hurt,

and I am inclined to assert myself with her and see if we can rebuild our relationship.

- However, when I believe 'Jill absolutely should not have betrayed my trust by telling Beryl my secret', I feel hurt and withdraw into myself, feeling sorry for myself and thinking that my relationship with Jill is over.

Make a commitment to belief change

Ask yourself: 'Which belief do I want to strengthen and which do I want to weaken, and why?'

After the questioning you have undertaken, it is very likely that you will decide that you wish to work to strengthen your conviction in your non-dogmatic preference and to weaken your conviction in your demand. You 'should' also be able to give coherent reasons why, based on your problematic feelings and behaviour and your goals for change.

Fiona's example
Question: 'Which belief do I want to strengthen and which do I want to weaken, and why?'
Answer:

- I want to strengthen my non-dogmatic preference, 'I would really have preferred it if Jill had not betrayed my trust by telling Beryl my secret, *but* unfortunately she doesn't have to do what I want her to do', because it is true, logical and will help me handle the situation with Jill in a healthier way, both emotionally and behaviourally.
- I want to weaken my rigid belief, 'Jill absolutely should not have betrayed my trust by telling Beryl my secret', because it is false, illogical and will interfere with me handling the situation with Jill in a healthier way, both emotionally and behaviourally.

8

Question your awfulizing belief and your anti-awfulizing belief

When questioning your awfulizing and anti-awfulizing beliefs, use the same three questions that you used to question your demands and non-dogmatic preferences: the empirical question, the logical question and the pragmatic question. Once you have done this you can then ask yourself which belief you want to strengthen and which you want to weaken, and why.

First, focus on your awfulizing belief and your anti-awfulizing belief alternative. Again write these down side by side, like this:

Awfulizing belief	Anti-awfulizing belief
It would be terrible if x happens (or does not happen).	It would be bad, but not terrible, if x happens (or does not happen).

Then move on to the three questions.

The empirical question

Ask yourself: 'Which of the following beliefs is true and which is false, and why?'

iB: My awfulizing belief..

....

rB: My anti-awfulizing belief ....

....

According to REBT theory, an awfulizing belief is false and an anti-awfulizing belief is true.

When you are holding an awfulizing belief, you believe the following:

1 Nothing could be worse.
2 The event in question is worse than 100 per cent bad.
3 No good could possibly come from this bad event.

If you think about it carefully, you will see that all three convictions are inconsistent with reality and that your anti-awfulizing belief is true, since this is made up of the following ideas:

1 Things could always be worse.
2 The event in question is less than 100 per cent bad.
3 Good could come from this bad event.

Fiona's example

Question: 'Which of the following beliefs is true and which is false, and why?'

- *Awfulizing belief:* 'It is terrible that Jill betrayed my trust by telling Beryl my secret.'
- *Anti-awfulizing belief:* 'It is bad that Jill betrayed my trust by telling Beryl my secret, *but* it isn't terrible that she did so.'

Answer: 'My anti-awfulizing belief is true and my awfulizing belief is false.'

- I can prove that having my trust betrayed by Jill is bad, but I can also prove that worse things could happen to me than that. I can also prove that good can come out of this experience. If it were true that having my trust betrayed in this way was awful, then nothing could be worse than this and no good could ever possible come from it. This is obviously not the case.

The logical question

Ask yourself: 'Which of the following beliefs is logical and which is illogical, and why?'

iB: My awfulizing belief ....

....

rB: My anti-awfulizing belief ....

....

According to REBT theory your awfulizing belief is illogical, while your anti-awfulizing belief is logical. Your awfulizing belief is based on the same evaluation of badness as your anti-awfulizing belief, but you transform this as follows:

> It would be very bad if 'A' happened ... and therefore it would be terrible.

Your awfulizing belief has two components. The first – 'It would be very bad if "A" happened' – is non-extreme, while the second – 'and therefore it would be terrible' – is extreme. As such, your awfulizing belief is illogical, since one cannot logically derive something extreme from something that is not extreme. The template in Figure 3 illustrates this.

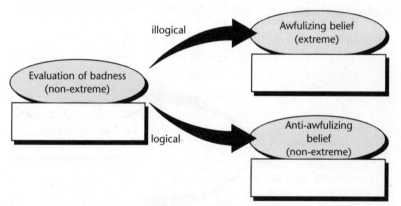

Figure 3 Your awfulizing and anti-awfulizing beliefs

Your anti-awfulizing belief is as follows:

> It would be very bad if 'A' happened ... but it would not be terrible.

Your anti-awfulizing belief is logical, since both parts are non-extreme, and thus the second component logically follows from the first. The template in Figure 3 illustrates this.

Fiona's example
Question: 'Which of the following beliefs is logical and which is illogical, and why?'

- *Awfulizing belief:* 'It is terrible that Jill betrayed my trust by telling Beryl my secret.'
- *Anti-awfulizing belief:* 'It is bad that Jill betrayed my trust by telling Beryl my secret, *but* it isn't terrible that she did so.'

Answer: 'My anti-awfulizing belief is logical and my awfulizing belief is illogical.'

- My awfulizing belief is based on the same evaluation of badness as my anti-awfulizing belief, but this is transformed, as we can see: 'It is bad that Jill betrayed my trust by telling Beryl my secret, and therefore it is terrible that she did so.' Thus, it has two components. The first ('It is bad that Jill betrayed my trust by telling Beryl my secret') is non-extreme, while the second ('and therefore it is terrible that she did so') is extreme. As such, my awfulizing belief is illogical, since in logic one cannot derive something extreme from something that is not extreme.
- On the other hand, my anti-awfulizing belief is logical, since both parts are non-extreme, and thus the second component logically follows from the first. This can be clearly shown in Figure 4.

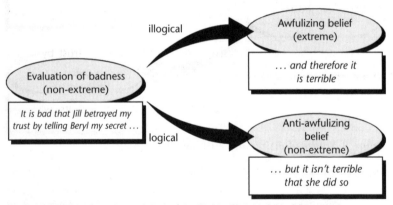

Figure 4 Why Fiona's awfulizing belief is illogical and her anti-awfulizing belief is logical

The pragmatic question

Ask yourself: 'Which of the following beliefs leads to largely healthy results and which leads to largely unhealthy results, and why?'

iB: My awfulizing belief ....

....

rB: My anti-awfulizing belief ....

....

MARK YOU WRENE & WILL MARRY ME . ♡

You need to acknowledge that your awfulizing belief leads to unhealthy results for you, while your anti-awfulizing belief leads to healthier results. Write down the consequences of holding both beliefs and refer, if necessary, to the section where I discussed 'iB–C' and 'rB–new C' connections, on p. 46.

Fiona's example
Question: 'Which of the following beliefs leads to largely healthy results and which leads to largely unhealthy results, and why?'
- *Awfulizing belief:* 'It is terrible that Jill betrayed my trust by telling Beryl my secret.'
- *Anti-awfulizing belief:* 'It is bad that Jill betrayed my trust by telling Beryl my secret, *but* it isn't terrible that she did so.'

Answer:
- My awfulizing belief will lead largely to unhealthy results, while my anti-awfulizing belief will lead to healthy results.
- My awfulizing belief, like my rigid demand, will lead me to feel hurt about Jill's betrayal of me. This will lead me to withdraw from her and regard our friendship as being over. My anti-awfulizing belief, on the other hand, like my non-dogmatic preference, will lead me to feel sorrowful, but not hurt, about Jill's betrayal. I will then be more likely to talk about my feelings with her and try to repair our relationship.

Make a commitment to belief change

Ask yourself: 'Which belief do I want to strengthen and which do I want to weaken, and why?'

After the questioning you have undertaken, you 'should' decide that you wish to work to strengthen your conviction in your anti-awfulizing belief and to weaken your conviction in your awfulizing belief. You 'should' also be able to give coherent reasons why, based on your problematic feelings and behaviour and your goals for change.

Fiona's example
Question: 'Which belief do I want to strengthen and which do I want to weaken, and why?'
Answer:

- I want to strengthen my anti-awfulizing belief, 'It is bad that Jill betrayed my trust by telling Beryl my secret, *but* it isn't terrible that she did so', because it is true, logical and will help me handle the situation with Jill in a healthier way, both emotionally and behaviourally.

- I want to weaken my awfulizing belief, 'It is terrible that Jill betrayed my trust by telling Beryl my secret', because it is false, illogical and will interfere with me handling the situation with Jill in a healthier way, both emotionally and behaviourally.

9

Question your LFT belief and your HFT belief

When questioning your low frustration tolerance (LFT) and high frustration tolerance (HFT) beliefs, again use the tripartite questioning approach: the empirical question, the logical question and the pragmatic question. Once you have done this, again ask yourself which belief you want to strengthen and which you want to weaken, and why.

Begin by focusing on your LFT belief and your HFT belief alternative. Again write these down side by side, like this:

LFT belief	HFT belief
I could not bear it if x happens (or does not happen).	It would be difficult to bear if x happens (or does not happen), but I could bear it and it would be worth it to me to do so.

Then move on to the three questions.

The empirical question

Ask yourself: 'Which of the following beliefs is true and which is false, and why?'

iB: My LFT belief ....

....

rB: My HFT belief ....

....

According to REBT theory, an HFT belief is true and an LFT belief is false.

When you are holding an LFT belief, you believe *at the time* the following:

1 I will die or disintegrate if the frustration or discomfort continues to exist.
2 I will lose the capacity to experience happiness if the frustration or discomfort continues to exist.

Step and back and see that these convictions are inconsistent with reality and that your HFT belief is true, since this is made up of the following ideas:

1 I will struggle if the frustration or discomfort continues to exist, but I will neither die nor disintegrate.
2 I will not lose the capacity to experience happiness if the frustration or discomfort continues to exist, although this capacity will be temporarily diminished.
3 The frustration or discomfort is worth tolerating.

Fiona's example

Question: 'Which of the following beliefs is true and which is false, and why?'

- *LFT belief:* 'I can't bear it that Jill betrayed my trust by telling Beryl my secret.'
- *HFT belief:* 'It is hard for me to put up with Jill betraying my trust by telling Beryl my secret, *but* I can tolerate it and it is worth it to me to do so.'

Answer: 'My HFT belief is true and my LFT is false.'

- I can prove that I can put up with Jill betraying my trust even though it is difficult for me to do so. I haven't lost the capacity to enjoy myself and I can survive the shock. I can also prove it is worth it for me to tolerate this betrayal. I would like to repair my relationship with Jill if I can, and believing that it is worth it for me to tolerate her behaviour will give me a chance to put things right between us if this is possible.
- If I couldn't tolerate Jill betraying my trust then I would disintegrate or lose the capacity for happiness. Neither is the case even if I believe it to be so.

The logical question

Ask yourself: 'Which of the following beliefs is logical and which is illogical, and why?'

iB: My LFT belief....:...

....

rB: My HFT belief ....

....

According to REBT theory your LFT belief is illogical, while your HFT belief is logical. Your LFT belief is based on the same idea of struggle as your HFT belief, but you transform this as follows:

It would be difficult for me to tolerate it if 'A' happened ... and therefore it would be intolerable.

Your LFT has two components. The first – 'It would be difficult for me to tolerate it if "A" happened' – is non-extreme, while the second – 'and therefore it would be intolerable' – is extreme. As such your LFT belief is illogical, since one cannot logically derive something extreme from something that is not extreme. The template in Figure 5 illustrates this.

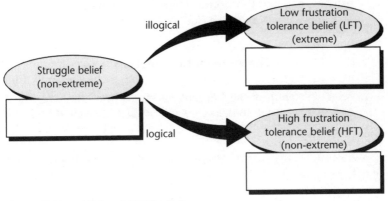

Figure 5 Your LFT and HFT beliefs

Your HFT belief is as follows:

> It would be difficult for me to tolerate it if 'A' happened ... but I can tolerate it and it is worth it to me to do so.

Your HFT belief is logical, since both parts are non-extreme and thus the second component logically follows from the first. Again, the template in Figure 5 illustrates this.

Fiona's example

Question: 'Which of the following beliefs is logical and which is illogical, and why?'

- *LFT belief:* 'I can't bear it that Jill betrayed my trust by telling Beryl my secret.'
- *HFT belief:* 'It is hard for me to put up with Jill betraying my trust by telling Beryl my secret, *but* I can tolerate it and it is worth it to me to do so.'

Answer: 'My HFT belief is logical and my LFT belief is illogical.'

- My LFT belief is based on the same sense of struggle as my HFT belief, but this is transformed, as we can see: 'It is hard for me to put up with Jill betraying my trust by telling Beryl my secret and therefore I can't bear it.' Thus it has two components. The first – 'It is hard for me to put up with Jill betraying my trust by telling Beryl my secret' – is non-extreme, while the second – 'and therefore I can't bear it' – is extreme. As such, my LFT belief is illogical, since in logic one cannot derive something extreme from something that is not extreme.
- On the other hand, my HFT belief is logical, since both parts are non-extreme, and thus the second component logically follows from the first. This is clearly shown in Figure 6.

The pragmatic question

> Ask yourself: 'Which of the following beliefs leads to largely healthy results and which leads to largely unhealthy results, and why?'
>
> iB: My LFT belief..
>
> ....
>
> rB: My HFT belief..
>
> ....

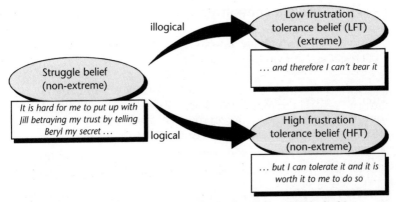

Figure 6 Why Fiona's LFT belief is illogical and her HFT belief is logical

You need to acknowledge that your LFT belief leads to unhealthy results for you, while your HFT belief leads to healthier results. Write down the consequences of holding both beliefs and refer again, if necessary, to the section on 'iB–C' and 'rB–new C' connections, on p. 46.

Fiona's example

Question: 'Which of the following beliefs leads to largely healthy results and which to largely unhealthy results, and why?'

- *LFT belief:* 'I can't bear it that Jill betrayed my trust by telling Beryl my secret.'
- *HFT belief:* 'It is hard for me to put up with Jill betraying my trust by telling Beryl my secret, *but* I can tolerate it and it is worth it to me to do so.'

Answer:

- My LFT belief will lead largely to unhealthy results, while my HFT belief will lead to healthy results.
- My LFT belief, like my rigid demand and my awfulizing belief, will lead me to feel hurt about Jill's betrayal of me and will lead me to withdraw from her and regard our friendship as being over. My HFT belief, on the other hand, like my non-dogmatic preference and my anti-awfulizing belief, will lead me to feel sorrowful, but not hurt, about Jill's betrayal. I will then be more likely to talk about my feelings with her and try to repair our relationship.

Make a commitment to belief change

Ask yourself: 'Which belief do I want to strengthen and which do I want to weaken, and why?'

After the questioning you have undertaken, you 'should' decide that you wish to work to strengthen your conviction in your HFT belief and to weaken your conviction in your LFT belief. You 'should' also be able to give coherent reasons why, based on your problematic feelings and behaviour and your goals for change.

Fiona's example
Question: 'Which belief do I want to strengthen and which do I want to weaken, and why?'
Answer:

- I want to strengthen my HFT, 'It is hard for me to put up with Jill betraying my trust by telling Beryl my secret, *but* I can tolerate it and it is worth it to me to do so', because it is true, logical and will help me handle the situation with Jill in a healthier way, both emotionally and behaviourally.

- I want to weaken my LFT, 'I can't bear it that Jill betrayed my trust by telling Beryl my secret', because it is false, illogical and will interfere with me handling the situation with Jill in a healthier way, both emotionally and behaviourally.

10

Question your self-depreciation belief and your self-acceptance belief

As I discussed in Chapter 2, hurt can involve self-depreciation. When it does, then you need to question your self-depreciation (your self-acceptance beliefs), again using the three questions I discussed in the previous chapters: the empirical question, the logical question and the pragmatic question. As before, once you have done this, again ask yourself which belief you want to strengthen and which you want to weaken, and why.

Focus on your self-depreciation belief and the self-acceptance belief alternative. Write these down side by side, like this:

Self-depreciation belief	Self-acceptance belief
If x happens (or does not happen), I am no good.	If x happens (or does not happen), it does not prove that I am no good. Rather, I am a fallible human being, a complex mixture of good, bad and neutral.

Then move on to the three questions.

The empirical question

Ask yourself: 'Which of the following beliefs is true and which is false, and why?'

iB: My self-depreciation belief ....

....

rB: My self-acceptance belief ....

....

According to REBT theory, a self-acceptance belief is true and a self-depreciation belief is false.

When you are holding a self-depreciation belief, you believe *at the time* the following:

1 You can legitimately be given a single global rating that defines your essence, and your worth as a person is dependent upon conditions that change (e.g. your worth goes up when you do well and goes down when you don't do well).
2 You can be rated on the basis of one of your aspects.

If you stand back, you will see that these convictions are inconsistent with reality and that your self-acceptance belief is true, since this is made up of the following ideas:

1 You cannot legitimately be given a single global rating that defines your essence, and your worth, as far as you have it, is not dependent upon conditions that change (e.g. your worth stays the same whether or not you do well).
2 It makes sense to rate discrete aspects of you, but it does not make sense to rate the whole of you on the basis of these discrete aspects.

Fiona's example

Question: 'Which of the following beliefs is true and which is false, and why?'

- *Self-depreciation belief:* 'Jill betraying my trust and telling Beryl my secret proves that I am not worth much.'
- *Self-acceptance belief:* 'Jill betraying my trust and telling Beryl my secret does not prove that I am not worth much. I am the same fallible human being whether Jill betrayed my trust or not. My worth is not dependent on her behaviour.'

Answer:

- My self-acceptance belief is true and my self-depreciation belief is false.
- I can prove that I am the same fallible human being whether Jill betrayed my trust or not. I am far too complex to be defined by one experience, and my fallibility is fixed and does not depend on what happens to me. So when I say that Jill betraying my trust by telling Beryl my secret proves that I am not worth much I am wrong, since this is inconsistent with reality.

The logical question

Ask yourself: 'Which of the following beliefs is logical and which is illogical, and why?'

iB: My self-depreciation belief ....

....

rB: My self-acceptance belief ....

....

According to REBT theory your self-depreciation belief is illogical, while your self-acceptance belief is logical.

When you hold a self-depreciation belief, this belief is based on the same idea as your self-acceptance belief – in both you acknowledge that it is bad if 'A' happens – but you transform it as follows:

'A' is bad ... and therefore I am bad.

Thus, your self-depreciation belief has two components. The first – '"A" is bad' – is an evaluation of a part of your experience, while the second – 'and therefore I am bad' is an evaluation of the whole of your 'self'. As such, you are making the illogical part–whole error, where the part is deemed illogically to define the whole.

Your self-acceptance belief is as follows:

'A' is bad, but this does not mean that I am bad. I am a fallible human being even though 'A' happened.

Your self-acceptance belief is logical because it shows that your 'self' is complex and incorporates a bad event. Thus, in holding your self-acceptance belief, you avoid making the part–whole error.

Fiona's example

Question: 'Which of the following beliefs is logical and which is logical/ illogical, and why?'

- *Self-depreciation belief:* 'Jill betraying my trust and telling Beryl my secret proves that I am not worth much.'
- *Self-acceptance belief:* 'Jill betraying my trust and telling Beryl my secret does not prove that I am not worth much. I am the same fallible human being whether Jill betrayed my trust or not. My worth is not dependent on her behaviour.'

Answer:

- My self-acceptance belief is logical and my self-depreciation belief is illogical. Jill betraying my trust is bad and that constitutes an evaluation of one experience. It is therefore part of my life, albeit a small part. To say that I am not worth much because this happened to me is illogical, because in saying this I am stating that one experience can define me as a person. In doing this I am making the part–whole error.
- On the other hand, when I say that Jill's behaviour does not make me worth less and that I am the same fallible human being whether or not she betrayed me, this is logical, because in saying this I am recognizing that my self incorporates this experience and is not defined by it. I therefore avoid making the part–whole error.

The pragmatic question

Ask yourself: 'Which of the following beliefs leads to largely healthy results and which leads to largely unhealthy results, and why?'

iB: My self-depreciation belief ....

....

rB: My self-acceptance belief ....

....

You need to acknowledge that your self-depreciation belief leads to unhealthy results for you, while your self-acceptance belief leads to healthier results. Write down the consequences of holding both beliefs, and if necessary refer once again to the section on 'iB–C' and 'rB–new C' connections, discussed on p. 46.

Fiona's example

Question: 'Which of the following beliefs leads to largely healthy results and which leads to largely unhealthy results, and why?'

- *Self-depreciation belief:* 'Jill betraying my trust and telling Beryl my secret proves that I am not worth much.'
- *Self-acceptance belief:* 'Jill betraying my trust and telling Beryl my secret does not prove that I am not worth much. I am the same fallible human being whether Jill betrayed my trust or not. My worth is not dependent on her behaviour.'

Answer:
- My self-depreciation belief will lead largely to unhealthy results, while my self-acceptance belief will lead to healthy results.
- My self-depreciation belief will lead me to feel hurt about Jill's betrayal of me and will lead me to withdraw from her and regard our friendship as being over. My self-acceptance belief, on the other hand, will lead me to feel sorrowful, but not hurt, about Jill's betrayal. I will then be more likely to talk about my feelings with her and try to repair our relationship.

Make a commitment to belief change

Ask yourself: 'Which belief do I want to strengthen and which do I want to weaken, and why?'

After the questioning you have undertaken, you 'should' decide that you wish to work to strengthen your conviction in your self-acceptance belief and to weaken your conviction in your depreciation belief. You 'should' also be able to give coherent reasons why, based on your feelings of hurt and your goals for change.

Fiona's example
Question: 'Which belief do I want to strengthen and which do I want to weaken, and why?'

Answer:
- I want to strengthen my self-acceptance belief, 'Jill betraying my trust and telling Beryl my secret does not prove that I am not worth much. I am the same fallible human being whether Jill betrayed my trust or not. My worth is not dependent on her behaviour', because it is true, logical and will help me handle the situation with Jill in a healthier way, both emotionally and behaviourally.
- I want to weaken my self-depreciation, 'Jill betraying my trust and telling Beryl my secret proves that I am not worth much', because it is false, illogical and will interfere with me handling the situation with Jill in a healthier way, both emotionally and behaviourally.

11

Begin to work on your rational and irrational beliefs

In this chapter, I will teach you a number of techniques devised to help you strengthen your conviction in your rational beliefs and weaken your conviction in your irrational beliefs. You need to work at truly believing rational beliefs in the sense that they make a real difference to the way that you feel and how you act.

Why? Because just understanding that your rational beliefs are consistent with reality, logical and helpful to you is not sufficient to bring about change. This form of understanding is known as *intellectual insight*. When you have it, you say things such as 'I understand why my rational belief is rational, but I don't believe it yet' or 'I understand that my rational belief is rational up here' (referring to your head) 'but not down here' (referring to your gut). This type of insight is necessary to help you change your core and specific rational beliefs but not sufficient for you to do so.

The type of insight that does promote change is known by REBT therapists as *emotional insight*. If you have this type of insight, you say such things as, 'Not only do I believe it in my head, I feel it in my gut' and 'I really believe in my heart that my healthy belief is true, logical and helpful.' The real indicator of whether you have emotional insight into your specific rational belief is that this belief leads to healthy emotions, constructive behaviour and realistic thinking. In this chapter, I will describe a number of techniques that are designed to help you to believe in your gut what you understand in your head.

The attack–response technique

This technique, which is sometimes called the zigzag technique, is based on the idea that you can strengthen your conviction in a rational belief by responding persuasively to attacks on this belief. There are a number of variations of this technique which I will briefly mention later. But first let me outline the main (written) version of the attack–response technique.

How to complete a written attack–response form

1 Write down your specific *rational* belief on a piece of paper.
2 Rate your present level of conviction in this belief on a 100-point scale, with 0 = no conviction and 100 = total conviction (i.e. 'I really believe this in my gut and it markedly influences my feelings and behaviour'). Write down this rating under your belief.
3 Write down an attack on this rational belief. Your attack may take the form of a doubt, reservation or objection to this rational belief. It should also contain an explicit irrational belief (e.g. demand, awfulizing belief, LFT belief or depreciation belief). Make this attack as genuinely as you can. The more it reflects what you believe, the better.
4 Respond to this attack as fully as you can. It is really important that you respond to each element of the attack. In particular, make sure that you respond to irrational belief statements and also to distorted or unrealistic inferences framed in the form of a doubt, reservation or objection to the rational belief. Do so as persuasively as possible, and write down your response.
5 Continue in this vein until you have answered all of your attacks and cannot think of any more. Make sure throughout this process that you are keeping the focus on the rational belief that you are trying to strengthen.
6 If you find this exercise difficult, make your attacks gently at first. Then, when you can respond to these attacks quite easily, begin to make the attacks more biting. Work in this way until you are making really strong attacks. When you make an attack, do so as if you really want to believe it. And when you respond, really throw yourself into it with the intention of demolishing the attack and of strengthening your conviction in your rational belief.
7 Don't forget that the purpose of this exercise is to strengthen your conviction in your rational belief, so it is important that you stop only when you have answered all of your attacks.

8 When you have answered all of your attacks, re-rate your level of conviction in your rational belief using the 0–100 scale as before. If you have succeeded at responding persuasively to your attacks, then this rating will have gone up appreciably.

Fiona's example

Here is how Fiona used the attack–response technique:

Rational belief: 'I would really have preferred it if Jill had not betrayed my trust by telling Beryl my secret, *but* unfortunately she doesn't have to do what I want her to do.'

[Conviction rating of rational belief = 25]

Attack: 'But it's not fair that she betrayed my trust and it absolutely should not be that way. She absolutely should have kept my secret.'

Response: 'Well, it may not be fair, but if there was a law of the universe that decreed that I must be treated fairly by Jill, then I would be treated fairly by her. That obviously didn't happen, and if I continue to tell myself that it absolutely should have done it won't change anything and I'll give myself the additional unfairness of hurt feelings.'

Attack: 'But you sound as if it doesn't matter that Jill betrayed your trust. Let's face it, it was terrible that she did so, particularly as she was at the time one of your best friends.'

Response: 'I am not saying that it doesn't matter that Jill betrayed my trust by telling Beryl my secret. It matters very much, but that isn't the same as saying that it's awful that she betrayed me. It's very bad, I admit, but awful? It's a long way from that. And Jill being a very good friend only increases the badness of what she did – it doesn't make it awful.'

Attack: 'But she promised you faithfully that she wouldn't tell anyone your secret and therefore she absolutely should have kept her word.'

Response: 'Yes, she did promise me faithfully that she would keep my secret, but that sadly does not mean that she had to do so. In the final analysis she is human and humans do at times break their promises. The fact that she was at the time one of my best friends does not change this grim reality.'

[Conviction rating of original rational belief = 70]

I mentioned earlier that there are a number of variations of the attack–response technique. Thus, you can record the dialogue and make sure that your response is more forceful in tone and language than your attack. You can also use the technique with a friend who can make increasingly biting attacks on your rational belief, encouraging you to respond effectively to these attacks. This is often called the devil's advocate technique.

Using rational-emotive imagery

Rational-emotive imagery (REI) is an imagery method designed to help you practise changing your *specific* irrational belief to its healthy equivalent while, at the same time, you use your imagination to focus on what you were most disturbed about in a *specific* situation in which you felt disturbed.

REI is based on the fact that you can use your imagery modality to help you get over your problems with hurt or, albeit unwittingly, to practise thinking unhealthily as you imagine a host of negative situations about which you make yourself feel hurt. In the latter case, when you think about a negative event and you make yourself feel hurt about it, you are likely to do so by imagining the event in your mind's eye and covertly rehearsing one or more irrational beliefs about the event. In this way, you literally practise making yourself feel hurt, and at the same time you end up strengthening your conviction in your irrational beliefs.

Fortunately, you can also use your mind's eye for constructive purposes. For instance, while imagining the same negative event as above, you can practise changing your feelings of hurt to those of sorrow, by changing your specific irrational beliefs to specific rational beliefs.

What follows is a set of instructions for using REI:

1 Take a situation in which you felt hurt and identify the aspect of the situation you were most hurt about.
2 Close your eyes and imagine the situation as vividly as possible. Focus on the adversity at 'A'.
3 Allow yourself to really experience the hurt feelings that you felt at the time, while still focusing intently on the 'A'.
4 Really experience your hurt for a moment or two and then change your emotional response to sorrow, which is the healthy negative alternative to hurt. While you do this, keep focusing intently on the adversity at 'A'. Do not change the intensity of your hurt; change it to sorrow, but keep the sorrow as strong as

your hurt. Keep experiencing your sorrow for about five minutes, all the time focusing on the 'A'. If you go back to your hurt feelings, bring your sorrow back.

5   At the end of five minutes, ask yourself how you changed your emotion.

6   Make sure that you changed your emotional response from hurt to sorrow by changing your specific irrational belief to its healthy alternative. If you did not do so (if, for example, you changed your emotion by changing the 'A' to make it less negative or neutral or by holding an indifference belief about the 'A'), do the exercise again, and keep doing this until you have changed your hurt to sorrow only by changing your specific unhealthy belief to its healthy alternative.

Fiona's example

1   Fiona chose the situation where Jill told Beryl her secret and focused on the aspect that she felt most hurt about, which was Jill's betrayal of her trust.

2   Fiona closed her eyes and imagined Jill telling Beryl her secret, and focused on her sense of being betrayed by Jill.

3   Fiona made herself feel very hurt while focusing on Jill's betrayal.

4   Fiona kept feeling hurt for a few moments, but then changed her feelings to sorrow about being betrayed by Jill. Initially she had trouble doing this, but eventually managed to do so. She maintained the same intensity of sorrow as she had of hurt.

5   Fiona then asked herself how she managed to change her feelings of hurt about being betrayed by Jill to feelings of sorrow.

6   Fiona changed her feelings of hurt about being betrayed by Jill to feelings of sorrow by changing her demand that Jill absolutely should not have betrayed her to her non-dogmatic preference, whereby she recognized that she is not immune from such betrayal, although she would much rather Jill had not betrayed her.

My final point about REI concerns how frequently you should practise it. I suggest that you practise it several times a day and aim for 30 minutes' daily practice (when you are not doing any other therapy homework). You might practise it more frequently and for a longer period of time when you are about to face a negative situation about which you are likely to feel hurt. When you are doing other therapy homework, 15 minutes' daily REI practice will suffice.

Teaching your rational beliefs to others

Another way of strengthening your conviction in your rational beliefs is to teach them to others. I am not suggesting that you play the role of therapist to friends and relatives, nor am I suggesting that you foist these ideas on people who are not interested in discussing them. Rather, I am suggesting that you teach rational beliefs to people who hold the alternative irrational beliefs and are interested in hearing what you have to say on the subject. When you do this, and in particular when the other person argues with your viewpoint in defending their position, you get the experience of responding to their arguments with persuasive arguments of your own, and in doing so you strengthen your conviction in your own rational beliefs. I suggest that you do this after you have developed competence in using the written attack–response technique discussed earlier, since the back-and-forth discussion which often ensues when you attempt to teach rational beliefs to others is reminiscent of this technique.

Fiona's example
Fiona had developed a fair measure of success in developing her rational belief about being betrayed by Jill when she met up with her friend Karen, who had just been betrayed by someone at work whom she trusted. Karen held a similar irrational belief about being betrayed, and Fiona attempted to teach Karen rational thinking about her own betrayal. While this did not prove successful, at least in the short term – Karen clung tenaciously to the idea that her work colleague absolutely should not have treated her in the way that she did – Fiona found the experience very valuable in that she could see clearly the false, illogical and unhelpful arguments Karen used to defend her irrational belief. In coming up with rational counter-arguments to Karen's points, Fiona developed greater conviction in her own rational beliefs about being betrayed by Jill.

Use of rational self-statements

Once you have developed your specific rational beliefs, you can develop shorthand versions of these beliefs which you can write down on a small card or, as one of my clients does, type them into the message folder of your mobile phone and review them periodically. Such review is especially useful when you are about to face an adversity and while you are actually facing one, assuming that it is feasible to glance at your rational message. You can also repeat these self-statements to yourself in a forceful, persuasive manner. When you repeat such rational self-statements, do so mindfully. Mindless repetition will have no impact on your feelings or behaviour.

Fiona's example

Fiona constructed the following rational self-statements, which helped her to increase her conviction in developing her rational beliefs about being betrayed by Jill:

- 'I'm not immune from Jill's betrayal even though I'd really like to be.'
- 'Jill's behaviour is reprehensible, but it's not the end of the world.'
- 'My worth isn't dependent on the way Jill has treated me.'
- 'I can bear Jill's betrayal of me and it's worth it to me to do so.'

Rehearsing your rational beliefs

Rehearse your rational beliefs while acting and thinking in ways that are consistent with these beliefs.

Perhaps the most powerful way of strengthening your rational belief is to rehearse it while facing the relevant adversity at 'A' and while acting and thinking in ways that are consistent with this rational belief. When all these systems are working together in sync and you keep them in sync repeatedly, you maximize your chances of strengthening your conviction in your rational beliefs.

Conversely, refrain from acting and thinking in ways that are consistent with your old irrational belief. This will be difficult for you, because you are used to acting and thinking in unconstructive ways when your irrational belief is activated. However, if you monitor your belief, your behaviour and your subsequent thinking, and respond constructively to all three when you identify them, then you will go against your tendency to evaluate yourself, others and/or the world in rigid and extreme terms (belief), to act self-defeatingly (behaviour) and to think unrealistically (subsequent thinking). If you do this successfully then you will gain valuable experience at weakening your conviction in your irrational beliefs and strengthening your conviction in your rational beliefs.

You need to set yourself homework tasks designed to help you to do the above. In doing so, it is important for you to acknowledge the following:

- You may have been employing a number of safety-seeking strategies designed to help you avoid facing adversities or protect yourself psychologically if you do have to face these adversities. Continued use of these strategies while you are endeavouring to change your irrational beliefs will undermine your attempts to do so. So, identify these safety-seeking strategies (which are largely behavioural and thinking in nature and can often be subtle and difficult to spot) and question the irrational beliefs that often underpin them, so that you can face the adversities fairly and squarely while rehearsing your developing rational beliefs and while acting and thinking in ways that are not safety-seeking in purpose.

- You will not experience a change in your unhealthy hurt feelings until after much integrated practice at holding to your rational beliefs and acting and thinking in ways that are consistent with these beliefs. Thus, emotional change tends to lag behind behavioural change and thinking change. If you understand this, then you will persist at changing your thinking and behaviour and will not get discouraged when your hurt feelings take longer to change.

- It is important that you face negative events about which you feel hurt, so that you can practise your rational beliefs and the constructive thinking and acting that stem from these beliefs. As you do so, face events that pose a challenge to your developing rational beliefs and related thoughts and behaviour, but which you do not find overwhelming for you at that time.

Fiona's example

To help herself act and think in ways consistent with her rational belief and refrain from acting and thinking in ways consistent with her irrational belief, Fiona first listed these behaviours and thoughts under their respective headings, as follows:

Rational belief

'I would really have preferred it if Jill had not betrayed my trust by telling Beryl my secret, *but* unfortunately she doesn't have to do what I want her to do. It's bad that she betrayed me, but not terrible!'

Actions consistent with my rational belief

- Telling Jill that I felt sorrowful when she told Beryl my secret and that I wished she hadn't done that.
- Asking Jill for an explanation for her behaviour.
- Telling my friends that I felt sorrowful about Jill's behaviour and stating to them that it was bad that she acted in that way, but not terrible.
- Correcting their irrationalities about the way I was treated.

Subsequent thoughts consistent with my rational belief

- Thinking of ways to express my sorrow to Jill, and to indicate that I want to repair our relationship.

Irrational belief

- 'Jill absolutely should not have betrayed my trust by telling Beryl my secret. It's terrible that she did.'

Actions consistent with my irrational belief

- Avoiding Jill.
- Telling my friends that I felt hurt about Jill's behaviour and stating to them that it was terrible that she acted in that way; agreeing with their irrationalities about the way I was treated.

Subsequent thoughts consistent with my irrational belief

- Thinking of ways of avoiding Jill.
- Going over in my mind the terrible nature of her behaviour towards me.

After making these two lists, Fiona resolved to rehearse her rational belief and think and act in the ways she had identified as being consistent with this belief, and did so whenever she could. She first imagined speaking to Jill before actually doing it, and as she did so, she rehearsed her rational belief.

Fiona also refrained from acting and thinking in ways she had identified as being consistent with her irrational belief. When she felt like acting and thinking in these ways, she used these urges to go back and question her irrational belief and remind herself why this belief is false, illogical and unproductive. She then reviewed her rational belief and the reasons why it is true, sensible and helpful to her.

In these ways, Fiona strengthened her conviction in her rational belief and weakened her conviction in her irrational belief.

After she had prepared for the encounter, as discussed above, Fiona spoke to Jill about her telling Beryl Fiona's secret. Jill at first denied this, but because Fiona kept her cool and indicated that she did not condemn Jill as a person, but was bitterly disappointed with her behaviour, Jill then admitted telling Beryl, claiming that she did not realize that it was a secret. After some discussion, Fiona and Jill agreed to differ on this issue and are still on friendly terms, although not as close as they once were. Fiona is sad about this, but pleased that she has some contact with Jill.

After using the methods described in this part of the book, Fiona now feels sorrowful, but not hurt, about this episode. As a consequence, she thinks about it far less frequently than she once did. As I mentioned above, Fiona and Jill are on friendly terms, but Fiona does not plan to confide in Jill again until they fully repair their relationship, if indeed they do so.

12

Question your inferences

When you feel hurt you tend to feel hurt about certain things that have happened to you or that you think have happened to you. I discussed the inferences that you make at 'A' when you feel hurt in Chapter 2. In addition, when you feel hurt you tend to think in certain ways, and these inferences can be best seen as thinking consequences ('C') of your hurt-based irrational beliefs.

These inferences may be accurate or distorted, and need to be questioned. In this chapter, I will begin by helping you to question your inferences at 'C', which tend to be highly distorted and skewed.

Questioning your thinking consequences at 'C'

Once you have successfully challenged your irrational beliefs, you are in a position to stand back and consider the truth of your hurt-derived inferences at 'C'. Feeling sorrowful, but not hurt, will help you to be objective about your hurt-derived inferences.

When challenging your hurt-derived inferences, ask yourself these useful questions:

1 How realistic is my thinking?
2 How else can I view this?
3 How likely is it to be true?
4 If I described my inference to someone I trust to give me an objective opinion about it, what would this person say to me?
5 If someone in the same situation told me he or she had this inference, what would I say to them about the validity of their inference?
6 Would 12 objective judges agree with my inference?
7 If not, what inference would these 12 objective judges make instead?

8 What data do I need to gather to check the validity of my inference, and how reliable would these data be?

Fiona's example
Once Fiona had gone through the process of assessing her specific 'ABC' and challenged her irrational beliefs and formed rational beliefs, she revisited her hurt-derived inferences and questioned the validity of these thinking consequences.

Inference 1: **All my friends betray me in the end.**
Question: How realistic is my thinking here?
Response: This is not true. I can think of many friends who have never betrayed me. In fact, most of my friends have never betrayed me. While one or two have betrayed me over the years, most of my friends have been trustworthy.

Inference 2: **Everyone will find out about my secret.**
Question: How else can I view this?
Response: I can stand back and think that while a number of friends may find out that I have met a man, it's unlikely that everyone will. Meeting a man is hardly unusual behaviour and unlikely to be of great interest to all. It is not as if I don't meet men. I do, and while I think this one may be special – and that is why I asked Jill to keep it a secret – it is not out of character for me to have dates with men. So when I stand back at look at things, it is realistic to say that while some of my friends will find out about this, not all will! After all, not all my friends know one another.

Inference 3: **I will become a laughing stock.**
Question: If someone in the same situation as me told me he or she had this inference, what would I say to them about the validity of the inference?
Response: I would say of course they wouldn't! Even if all my friends do know that I have met a man, it is hardly likely that I will become a laughing stock. Why should I? It is not unusual behaviour for women in my friendship group to go out with men. When I go through my friends one by one, I cannot actually think of one who would turn a hair. They would be interested about him, but that would be natural. But a laughing stock? Certainly not!

Reconsider your 'A'

You will recall that in Chapter 5 I asked you to identify what you felt most hurt about in the episode that you chose to analyse. I also urged you to assume that it was true that, for example, the other person had mistreated you. I encouraged you to do this in order to identify the irrational beliefs that lay at the core of your hurt. If you had questioned your inference of mistreatment before this step, then you might have stopped feeling hurt if you concluded that the other person had not, in fact, treated you badly.

However, if you had managed to overcome your feelings of hurt by doing so, then you would have done this without identifying, challenging and changing the irrational beliefs that really determined your hurt feelings. In REBT, we call this changing 'A' rather than changing 'B'. If you had bypassed your irrational beliefs at this point, you would still be vulnerable to feeling hurt about the event in question if you later thought that your inference had been correct in the first place. In addition, if you had challenged your 'A' without first questioning your irrational beliefs, this challenge would have been coloured by the ongoing existence of these irrational beliefs and would thus not be objective.

You are in a much better position, therefore, to question your inference at 'A' that the other person has mistreated you, for example, *after* you have challenged and changed your irrational beliefs. Doing so will help you to be more objective in your questioning of your 'A'. Putting this differently: feeling sorrowful, but not hurt, will help you to stand back and take an objective view about your 'A', while feeling hurt will interfere with your objectivity.

When you come to challenge your inference at 'A', ask yourself the same questions that I outlined on p. 83.

Fiona's example

Feeling sorrow rather than hurt in the episode that she chose to analyse helped Fiona to be objective about how Jill 'betrayed my trust by revealing my secret'. She still considered Jill was wrong to reveal her secret, but on second thoughts considered that 'betrayal' was too strong a word for what Jill did. After all, Fiona reasoned, 'Jill was thrilled when I told her about my news and may not have registered that I really wanted her to keep it secret. Indeed, the fact that I was thrilled myself may have meant that I may not have stressed that I really wanted her to keep my news to herself.'

Fiona acknowledged that she would not have been able to think with such objectivity when she was feeling hurt. She recognized, therefore, the value of first addressing the irrational beliefs that underpinned her hurt feelings before then re-examining inferences from the perspective of sorrow-based rational beliefs.

In the final part of the book, I will draw upon the skills I have taught you in this part to help you become less prone to hurt – if hurt is indeed a pervasive problem for you.

Part 3

BECOME LESS PRONE TO HURT

This final part of the book is particularly relevant if hurt is a pervasive problem for you. If this is the case, you may well find yourself experiencing hurt in many of your relationships. As such, read the following very carefully and resolve to act on my suggestions. Just reading them is not enough: you have to act on them and do so repeatedly if you are to succeed at becoming less prone to experiencing hurt.

If you are unsure whether or not you are particularly prone to hurt, consult pp. 21–2 in Chapter 2. If you are prone to hurt, put into practise the following, which are designed to help you become less prone to this painful and disturbed emotion:

1 Acknowledge that hurt is a problem for you and prepare to change.
2 Develop general sorrow-based rational beliefs.
3 Think and act in ways that are consistent with your general rational beliefs.
4 Question your role in others' mistreatment of you and change accordingly.
5 Check for biases in viewing and making inferences about others' behaviour.
6 Understand others from their perspective.
7 Develop and rehearse a healthy philosophy of relationships.

Throughout this part of the book, many of the examples that I will use focus on dealing with being treated badly by others. This is for convenience only, and the points that I make apply equally to the entire range of inferences about which you may feel hurt and that I discussed in Chapter 2.

13

Acknowledge that hurt is a problem and prepare to change

Acknowledge that you are prone to hurt and that it is a problem for you

Once you have understood the nature of hurt (see Chapter 2 for a review), you have to do two things before you proceed. First, you have to decide whether you are prone to hurt; re-reading pp. 21–2 will be particularly helpful here. If you are, the second step is to decide whether being thus prone is a problem for you that you would like to change. With respect to this second point, take a sheet of paper and write down the advantages and disadvantages of experiencing hurt, from both a short-term and a long-term perspective. In doing so, review times when you have experienced hurt and remember what its consequences were. If you do this exercise thoroughly, you will, in all probability, see that the disadvantages of experiencing hurt clearly outweigh any advantages.

Once you have listed the advantages and disadvantages of feelings of hurt, you may find it helpful to question whether or not its advantages really are benefits, particularly from a long-term perspective. If you are unsure, ask yourself whether you would counsel somebody you care for to experience hurt for the reason that you see as an advantage. Even if there are some benefits, recognize that you may derive these from experiencing sorrow without incurring the costs of hurt. Thus, hurt may motivate you to re-evaluate the relationship you have with the person you consider acted badly towards you, but sorrow will do this as well, and more constructively. In this latter respect, you may find it useful to review the consequences of hurt and sorrow that I discussed in Chapters 2 and 3 respectively.

Take responsibility for being prone to hurt

You may accept that you are prone to hurt and see clearly that it is a problem for you which you would like to change, but unless you take responsibility for being prone to hurt, you will not be effective in becoming less prone to it. Taking responsibility for your feelings of hurt means fully acknowledging that while being treated badly and undeservedly by those close to you contributes to your feeling hurt, this behaviour does not and cannot on its own cause you to feel hurt. Rather, it is the irrational beliefs that you hold about this state of affairs that largely explain why you feel hurt. Taking responsibility for being prone to hurt means fully acknowledging that you hold such irrational beliefs in a variety of different situations and/or about a number of different people.

Assuming such responsibility is an important step in becoming less prone to hurt. Without taking this step you will continue to be prone to hurt feelings, because you will have done nothing to change the irrational beliefs that underpin your proneness.

Acknowledge that sorrow is the healthy alternative to hurt

Once you have taken responsibility for your proneness to feeling hurt and wish to overcome it, the next step is to set yourself an appropriate goal for change. It is no good working to overcome your feelings of hurt unless (1) you have a clear idea of what you are going to experience instead; and (2) this alternative emotion is acceptable to you. If either of these two conditions is absent, then you will make it much harder for yourself to become less prone to feeling hurt. Thus, if you cannot see any alternative to hurt you will tend to think that you are bound to experience it. If you see that sorrow is an alternative to feeling hurt but is not an acceptable one, then you will not work towards experiencing it.

Before you take this step, review Chapter 3, which is devoted to outlining the nature of sorrow. Then, when you are clear that you have understood why sorrow is healthy for you, take another sheet of paper and write down the advantages and disadvantages of experiencing this emotion, again from a short-term and a long-term perspective. In doing so, review those occasions when you experienced hurt, but this time imagine that you experienced sorrow instead (use the material in Chapter 3 if you get stuck). Particularly, focus on the consequences of this alternative emotion.

Once you have compiled this list, you will probably conclude that experiencing sorrow is a plausible and constructive alternative to experiencing hurt. You will probably see that the disadvantages of sorrow are not, in fact, disadvantages. Even if you still think that they are disadvantageous, by seeing the total picture you can recognize that such disadvantages are not stumbling blocks to working towards experiencing sorrow.

Make a commitment to feel sorrow rather than hurt

After you have fully understood that sorrow is the constructive alternative to feeling hurt, it is important that you make a commitment to work towards experiencing this emotion when you face a situation where, for example, others have treated you badly. You may find it helpful to make a written commitment to this effect and to review this every day. Also, you may consider telling a close friend that you are going to work towards experiencing sorrow rather than hurt, if you consider that this verbal commitment will help you to do the work necessary to achieve your goal.

Accept yourself for being prone to feeling hurt

One of the major obstacles to capitalizing on your commitment to become less prone to feeling hurt at this point may be your attitude of self-depreciation for being prone to hurt. When you do this, you rate your entire 'self' on the basis of this proneness. Doing so will distract you from working to overcome your hurt problem and will lead you to feel an unhealthy negative emotion, such as shame. Depreciating yourself for being prone to hurt has two main effects. It does nothing to make you any less prone to this destructive emotion, and it gives you two emotional problems for the price of one: your original hurt, and shame for experiencing such hurt.

If this applies to you, it is important that you work towards accepting yourself for being prone to feeling hurt. You do this by seeing that your proneness does not define your 'self' but is a part of your fallibility and complexity as a human being.

Accepting yourself for being prone to hurt will enable you to focus on the factors that make you thus prone, and will encourage you to do something constructive about it (like follow the guidelines in this part of the book) rather than resigning yourself to it. Self-acceptance, therefore, promotes constructive action and discourages passivity and resignation.

14

Develop general sorrow-based rational beliefs

Perhaps the most important step that you can take in becoming less prone to hurt is to develop a set of general rational beliefs to replace your hurt-based irrational beliefs. In the second part of this book, I showed you how to deal with specific episodes of hurt, and continuing to do this is important in developing more general sorrow-based rational beliefs.

Keep working on specific episodes of hurt

As I have just noted, in Part 2 of this book I outlined the steps that you need to take when working on specific episodes of hurt. In particular, I showed you how to identify what you were most hurt about and how to assess, challenge and change the irrational beliefs that under-pinned your situationally based feelings of hurt. I recommend that you do this as soon as you notice that you are making yourself hurt. Initially, you will need to do this on paper, but after much practice you will be able to do it in your head. You will also be more able to anticipate situations in which you are likely to make yourself feel hurt, and to deal productively with your hurt-related irrational beliefs before they take hold and lead to feelings of hurt.

Identify and make use of recurring patterns in your specific examples of hurt

Once you have worked through a number of specific examples of your hurt, you will be able to identify recurring patterns in these specific examples. Thus, you may find that your feelings of hurt are mainly related to your inference that someone close to you has betrayed your trust. If so, make a note of this theme and the people you think have betrayed your trust. Also, are your feelings of hurt ego-based or non ego-based?

Once you have identified recurring patterns in the specific episodes you have worked on, you can use this information in two main ways. First, you can utilize this information when you work to prevent the occurrence of hurt in vulnerable situations, and second, this information will be useful when you come to identify the general irrational beliefs that help to explain why you are prone to hurt.

Identify, challenge and change your general hurt-related irrational beliefs

General hurt-related irrational beliefs are irrational beliefs that are general in nature and account for your feelings of hurt across situations. While I will now give you some common examples of such beliefs, it is very important that you identify, challenge and change those irrational beliefs that are personal to you.

- 'People whom I have trusted must not betray that trust, and it is terrible when they do.'
- 'I must not be excluded by friends when others have been included. If I am, it proves that I am worthless.'
- 'When I do favours for people, they must reciprocate, and I can't bear it when they don't. Poor me!'
- 'People close to me must not forget events that are special to me. If they do, this means that they don't care for me and this proves that I am not worth caring about.'

Challenge your general irrational beliefs in the same way that you learned to challenge your specific irrational beliefs. Thus, take one of your general irrational beliefs and ask yourself the following questions:

- Is this belief true or false?
- Is this belief logical or illogical?
- Is this belief healthy or unhealthy?

At this point, you may find it beneficial to review the material on challenging specific irrational beliefs which can be found in

Chapters 7–10. Continue this line of questioning until you clearly understand that your general irrational beliefs are false, illogical and unconstructive.

Next, develop rational alternatives to the general irrational beliefs that you identified earlier. Personalize them as before. Here are the rational alternatives to the common examples of general irrational beliefs that I listed before:

- 'I really don't want people whom I have trusted to betray that trust, but sadly and regretfully that does not mean that they must not do so. It is very bad, but not terrible, when they do so.'

- 'I very much want to be included by friends when others have been included, but it is not essential that I am. If I am excluded that is bad, but it does not prove that I am worthless. My worth depends on me being alive and human and not on whether friends include me or not.'

- 'When I do favours for people, it is desirable, but not absolutely necessary, for them to reciprocate. When they don't do so, that is tough to bear, but I can bear it and it is worth bearing. I am not a poor person when this happens. Rather, it is a poor situation to be in.'

- 'It is very important to me that people close to me do not forget events that are special to me, but this does not mean that they must not do so. If they do forget, it does not follow that they don't care for me, but even if this is the case I am still worth caring about. My worth is not altered by whether or not people care for me.'

Once you have developed your general rational beliefs, question them in the same way as you questioned your general irrational beliefs. Do this until you clearly understand that your general rational beliefs are true, logical and constructive.

Now that you have done this, I suggest that you use the attack–response technique to deepen your conviction in your general rational beliefs (see pp. 74–5 for instructions concerning how to implement this technique).

Develop six broad sorrow-based rational philosophies

In the previous section I encouraged you to develop your own general rational beliefs. In this section, I will outline some general rational philosophies that will stand you in good stead and help you work on making yourself less prone to hurt feelings.

Accept that you are not immune from being treated badly by others

If you are particularly prone to non-ego hurt, it is important that you accept that you are not immune from being treated badly by others, no matter how close they are to you. In order to do this you have to revisit the following rule and carefully examine what it means:

> If you are fair to people then they will be fair to you, particularly if they are close to you.

If you look carefully at this rule, you will see that it attempts to describe what happens in the world. However, it is too general and is, in fact, wrong. A more accurate rule is probabilistic in nature, in that it makes a statement about what will happen in all probability but allows for exceptions. If we reformulate the above rule to make clear its probabilistic nature, we have the following:

> If you are fair to people then they will, in all probability, be fair to you, particularly if they are close to you.

Now, if we add in the bit which allows for exceptions, we have the following:

> If you are fair to people then they will, in all probability, be fair to you, particularly if they are close to you, *but it is not inevitable that they always will.*

However, it is still possible to believe the above rule and yet hold that it does not apply to you. We frequently go about our business believing that we have personal immunity from events that we easily acknowledge may well happen to other people. How often have you heard yourself or others say: 'I never thought that it would happen to me'? Sadly and regretfully, in all probability we are neither immune nor exempt from the possibility of bad things happening to us, no matter how much we do not deserve the bad things in question. We have no fairy godmother looking after us and God, if you believe in him or her, in all probability will not grant you such personal immunity. After all, why you rather than others? Accepting that we are not immune from unfair treatment at the hands of others, even from those towards whom we have always acted fairly, is a bitter pill to swallow, but you would be wise to swallow it if you want to become less prone to feelings of hurt in your life. So I strongly recommend that you fully accept, digest and use the following reformulated rule to guide you in your dealings with people.

> If you are fair to people then they will, in all probability, be fair to you, particularly if they are close to you, but it is not inevitable that they always will. I have no personal immunity from this rule, and thus I accept that, sadly and regretfully, people close to me can at times treat me unfairly, even though I have treated them well.

Accept yourself when others do treat you badly

If you are particularly prone to ego hurt, then it is important that you strive towards unconditional self-acceptance. Work on digesting the following points:

- As a human being you have great complexity and your worth as a person should reflect this. When you think you are more worthwhile if you are treated fairly by friends or less worthwhile if they treat you unfairly, then you are not doing justice to your complexity.
- When you rate yourself on the basis of what happens to you, you are making the part–whole error. This is where you use the event (e.g. when a friend excludes you) to judge your whole self (that you are worthless as a person). When you accept yourself you do not make the part–whole error because you acknowledge that whether or not your friend includes you only proves that you are the same person who was either included or excluded.
- Once you base your worth on how others treat you, you 'feel' temporarily good about yourself when you are treated well, but as soon as you are treated unfairly you will go back to 'feeling'

less worthwhile about yourself. However, if you accept yourself unconditionally, you are far less vulnerable in this respect.

If you would like to know a lot more about developing self-acceptance, then I suggest that you consult my book on the subject, *How to Accept Yourself* (Sheldon Press, 1999).

Develop an anti-awfulizing attitude towards undeserved treatment

Whether your feelings of hurt are ego-based or non ego-based, it is important that you take the horror, but not the badness, out of being treated in ways that you think are undeserved.

- Show yourself that being treated badly by others is bad, but certainly not the end of the world, unless you choose to view it in these terms.
- List the possible good that can come out of being treated badly. You may think that there is nothing to be gained from it, but you would be wrong. For example, being treated badly gives you the opportunity of handling such eventualities more healthily now and in the future. If others didn't treat you badly, you would not have the chance of developing resilience. Also, being treated badly may remind you of the fact that you may be wittingly or unwittingly treating others badly yourself. You may thus become more aware of your own negative impact on others and have the opportunity of correcting your own mistreatment of others.

If it were true that it is awful to be treated badly by others, then no good could possibly come out of this experience. Don't forget, though, that taking the horror out of undeserved treatment does not mean that you have to minimize the badness of such behaviour.

Tolerate the discomfort that occurs when others treat you badly

If you are particularly prone to non-ego hurt, then it is important that you strive to raise your tolerance for being treated badly. Work on digesting the following points:

- Show yourself that, while the discomfort that you are bound to feel when others treat you badly is tough to bear, it is definitely bearable. If it were unbearable then you could not bear it, no matter how you thought about it. If this were the case then you would die or disintegrate, even if you firmly believed that you could tolerate being treated badly by others. This is obviously not so, and thus being treated badly by others is not inherently unbearable. The problem resides in your attitude of LFT rather than in the bad treatment itself. This is actually very good news, since you can almost always change your own attitude whereas you don't have direct control of the behaviour of others.
- List reasons why it is worth tolerating the discomfort of being treated badly by others.
- List things that you can enjoy in life even though others have treated you badly.
- Write a short essay for your own children and/or for children in general, explaining to them why being treated badly by others is difficult to tolerate, but definitely bearable and worth bearing. Be as persuasive as you can be.

If you would like to know a lot more about developing high frustration tolerance, then I suggest that you consult a book that I wrote on the subject (with Jack Gordon), entitled *Beating the Comfort Trap* (Sheldon Press, 1993).

Accept others when they treat you badly, thus overcoming feelings of resentment

When you are prone to hurt you are also likely to feel resentment. It follows that if you want to become less prone to hurt, it would be useful for you to overcome your feelings of resentment. Resentment is a form of unhealthy anger that you feel towards someone you consider to have mistreated you in some way. More crucially, you believe

1 the person absolutely should not have treated you in this way;
2 the person is bad for doing so and needs to be punished; and
3 you need to gain revenge for being mistreated.

In order to overcome your feelings of resentment, you need to challenge and change the above irrational beliefs. First, you need to accept that, while you would much rather the other person did not mistreat you, sadly and regretfully there is no law of the universe that decrees that he or she must not act in that way.

Second, you need to distinguish between the person and his or her behaviour. Even if he (in this case) treated you badly, show yourself that his personhood is not defined by his behaviour. He is fallible and not bad. Viewing him as such does not condone or minimize the badness of his behaviour. Nor does it absolve him from assuming responsibility for his actions.

Third, see clearly that revenge will only increase the chances of you being mistreated in the future by the person concerned, since it is based on an 'eye for an eye' philosophy. If you take revenge on the person, he or she is more likely to feel the need to take revenge on you subsequently and this will only escalate mutual mistreatment. Instead, assert yourself firmly but respectfully, and check out your inferences as you do so!

If you do develop, practise and act on the above rational beliefs, you will overcome your feelings of resentment and become less prone to hurt as a result.

Surrender the 'poor me' attitude

If you are particularly prone to non-ego hurt then it is likely that you hold a 'poor me' attitude. In common parlance, you feel sorry for yourself. This is a difficult attitude to own up to, since we tend to feel ashamed about feeling sorry for ourselves. When we feel such shame, we will tend to deny that we hold the 'poor me' attitude.

So first, if you do feel sorry for yourself for being treated in an undeserving manner, you need to accept yourself for your feelings of self-pity. Show yourself that while these feelings and the behaviours that they lead to are unpleasant and unattractive, experiencing these feelings does not change you as a person. You are the same unique, fallible human being as you would be if you did not feel sorry for yourself. Remember that being fallible means that you are a complex mixture of good, bad and neutral features. So while feeling sorry for yourself may be a bad feature, you are not diminished for experiencing self-pity. It is bad, but you are not! If you need help with shame and self-acceptance, I suggest that you consult my two books on the subject (*Overcoming Shame*, 1997, and *How to Accept Yourself*, 1999, both Sheldon Press).

Once you have accepted yourself for holding the 'poor me' attitude, you are in a position to focus on this attitude and question it. Let's do that now.

When you hold the 'poor me' attitude, you believe that you are a poor person for being treated badly. While you may be correct in claiming that being badly treated by someone close to you places you in a poor situation, and particularly so if you have done nothing to deserve such treatment, you are not correct in concluding that you are a poor person for being in this poor situation. When you feel sorry *for yourself* and not just for the poor situation in which you find yourself, you are making the same part–whole error as you make when you depreciate yourself (see pp. 69–70). You make the part–whole error when you think (and let's suppose for the moment that you are correct in your interpretation) that you are in a poor situation and then define yourself as a poor person for being in this situation. This is obviously not the case. As a person you are very complex and cannot legitimately be defined by any situation in which you find yourself.

Thus, if you want to surrender the 'poor me' attitude, it is important that you refrain from making the part–whole error and recognize instead that whatever situation you are in – good, bad or neutral – you are the same complex non-poor person. By all means feel sorry *that* you are being treated badly, but do not feel sorry *for yourself* for being in this poor situation.

Defining yourself as a complex, non-poor person when you are in a poor situation, rather than a poor person, is perhaps the most important part of surrendering the 'poor me' attitude. However, you need to address other issues during the surrendering process, and I will discuss these issues more generally in the next chapter. They involve you thinking and acting in ways that are consistent with your developing rational beliefs.

15

Be consistent with your general rational beliefs

In Chapter 2, I noted the fact that when you hold general hurt-related irrational beliefs, these beliefs have an effect on the way that you subsequently tend to think and act. If you turn these tendencies into actualities, then you strengthen your conviction in these irrational beliefs and make yourself more prone to experience hurt.

In Chapter 3, on the other hand, I pointed out that when you hold sorrow-related general rational beliefs, these beliefs have a different and more constructive effect on the way that you subsequently tend to think and act. If you turn these tendencies into actualities, then you strengthen your conviction in these rational beliefs and make yourself less prone to experience hurt.

Following on from the above, I suggest that you:

1 Develop a list of the ways in which you tend to think and act once you feel hurt.
2 Notice times when you experience the tendency to think and act in the above ways and do not engage with these tendencies. Instead, use them as cues to go back to challenge the hurt-related irrational beliefs that spawned them.
3 Develop a list of the ways in which you would tend to think and act if you held sorrow-related irrational beliefs. These should be constructive alternatives to the thinking and action tendencies that you listed under Point 1 above.
4 Encourage yourself to think and act in ways that are consistent with the thinking and action tendencies that you listed under Point 3, once you have challenged your hurt-related irrational beliefs and have begun to hold the rational alternatives to these beliefs.

Thus, a powerful way of making yourself less prone to hurt is to practise developing your rational beliefs at the same time as you think and act in ways that reinforce such beliefs. If you hold sorrow-related rational beliefs but think and act in ways that are consistent with the hurt-related irrational beliefs, you will tend to go back to these beliefs and spoil the work that you are trying to do to make yourself less prone to hurt. Thus, guard against doing this.

Let's now consider the thinking and behaviour that will reinforce the rational beliefs that will help you be become less prone to hurt.

Think in ways that are consistent with your general rational beliefs

Let me stress again that once you have developed an appropriate set of rational beliefs about being mistreated by others, it is important that you think and act in ways that are consistent with these rational beliefs and forego thinking and acting in ways that are consistent with your hitherto irrational beliefs. This is a very important point. If you try to change your beliefs without changing your unconstructive behaviour and your subsequent distorted thinking, you will not, in the final analysis, change your beliefs. A return to old ways of behaviour and thinking is indeed a powerful but unintended way of practising the irrational beliefs that spawned them.

I will presently consider a number of constructive behaviours that stem from general sorrow-related rational beliefs about being badly treated by others. But first, I will consider the realistic forms of thinking that tend to follow these general rational beliefs. Practising these realistic forms of thinking will help you to deepen your conviction in your general rational beliefs.

View the other person's behaviour in context and without exaggeration

When you hold a general sorrow-based rational belief about being mistreated by others, this will help you to view their behaviour in context and without exaggeration. You can facilitate this type of realistic thinking by attempting to put yourself into the frame of reference of the other person or people, and trying to see the world through their eyes (see Chapter 18). If you are able to do this, such empathy may help you to put their behaviour into an understandable context, and in doing so you will tend to take the exaggeration out of your subsequent thinking. A similar effect will be produced if you ask yourself how an impartial jury might view their behaviour and the reasons for it.

See the other person not as malevolent, but as having complex motives

If you have been able to put yourself into the shoes of the relevant other person(s), as discussed above, you may also be able to acknowledge that they may have had a set of complex motives for their behaviour, and that while the effect of their behaviour may have been mistreatment of you, this may not have been their intention. Thus, your sorrow-based rational beliefs may help you to see the world in more complex ways than your irrational beliefs. The latter tend to restrict your vision so that all you see are malevolent motives behind people's behaviour. These will then tend to reinforce your irrational beliefs so that you end up getting trapped in a vicious circle. Seeing the complexity behind people's motives, by contrast, will help to reinforce your rational beliefs, and the resulting virtuous circle will help stop you seeing mistreatment where none occurred, or put such mistreatment into context when it did occur but was not intended.

See yourself as in a poor situation, not as a poor person

The irrational beliefs that underpin non-ego hurt lead you to feel sorry for yourself, as I discussed in Chapter 2. When you feel sorry for yourself you tend to think of yourself as alone, uncared for and misunderstood, and while doing so you think that this tends to define your place in the world rather than being restricted to the situation at hand. This type of thinking will then tend to reinforce the irrational beliefs that lead you to feel sorry for yourself in the first place.

Consequently, if you are to strengthen your sorrow-based rational beliefs, it is important that you acknowledge that being mistreated puts you in a poor situation but does not prove that you are a poor person. And if you do see yourself as alone, uncared for and misunderstood, make sure that you restrict this to the specific episode in question and do not over-generalize to this defining your enduring place in the world as a whole.

Think in a balanced way about past treatment from people

When you hold irrational beliefs about being mistreated, these beliefs lead you to look back at your life and see mainly poor treatment from others. Remember that irrational beliefs have a rigid quality and skew the way you see and remember things very much to the negative. When you practise your sorrow-based rational beliefs, it is important, therefore, to ensure that when you look back at your life you do so with realism. Look for, acknowledge and focus on times in your life when you were treated well by others, as well as badly. These will exist, and it is important that you find them, but only while you are looking at the world through the lens of your rational beliefs.

Think about how best to assert yourself

As I will presently show you, when you hold sorrow-based rational beliefs you will be much more likely to assert yourself with the person who has mistreated you than to sulk. These rational beliefs will also encourage you to think about how best to assert yourself with the person concerned. Thus, you will think about the person and judge how you might best put what you have to say, to maximize the chances that they will listen to you. Thinking in this way will help reinforce your rational beliefs.

Act in ways that are consistent with your general rational beliefs

There are two major forms of constructive behaviour that stem from general rational beliefs about (in this case) being mistreated by others.

Show that you accept the other person but dislike their behaviour

When you are feeling hurt about being mistreated and you talk about your experiences with others, you tend to denigrate the person or people who have mistreated you; even if you do not start out by doing so, you agree with the reactions of the people you are talking to when they themselves denigrate the other(s).

So when you are rehearsing your rational beliefs about being mistreated and discussing your experiences of being mistreated with others, show the people you are talking to that you accept the people who treated you badly as fallible human beings who have done the wrong thing, while also indicating that you dislike their treatment of you. And if they say that they disagree with you and that the person concerned is a bad person who absolutely should not have treated you this way, debate with them and give reasons for your rational beliefs. Your goal is not so much to persuade them to adopt your rational point of view as to rehearse this point of view so that you increase your conviction in it.

Maintain direct channels of communication with the other person

One of the main behaviours that accompanies hurt feelings is sulking. When you sulk, you withdraw from the person and demand internally that she (in this case) takes the first step in making amends to you, even if that person does not know what she has done to 'hurt' you. In doing so, you indirectly communicate to the person that you feel hurt. As sulking reinforces your hurt-creating irrational beliefs, it is important that you forego acting in such a way if you want to become less prone to hurt, even though sulking may have short-term advantages for you (see p. 89 for a discussion of this issue). The healthy alternative to sulking is direct, assertive communication. Such communication, in this context, involves you doing the following:

- Take responsibility for feeling sorrowful about being mistreated by the person.
- Tell the other person that you felt sorrowful about the way she treated you.

- Communicate clearly how you want the other person to treat you, but recognize that she did not have to treat you that way, and communicate that to her if appropriate.
- Ask the other person for an explanation of her mistreatment of you and respond without hurt (or anger) to what she says. Reiterate your preference, if necessary.
- Come to an agreement concerning her future behaviour towards you.

Committing yourself to direct assertive communication when people mistreat you, rather than sulking in the face of such behaviour, and acting consistently on that commitment is an important way to become less hurt-prone.

Deal with short-term gains

When you feel hurt and you tell people about how badly you have been treated by others, it is likely that you will receive a number of 'benefits' from doing so. These so-called gains are in the main short term in nature, but if you strive to achieve them they will serve to maintain your hurt feelings.

The antidote to these gains is talk which reflects your rational beliefs about the ways in which others have treated you.

Give up gain 1: Don't wallow in others' sympathy or self-pity

When you discuss your hurt feelings with others and tell them about the mistreatment you have received at the hands of someone, it is likely that you will gain their sympathy, at least initially. Sympathy from others is often based on an attitude of other-pity. Such people feel sorry for you, and this attitude may encourage you to feel sorry for yourself. Indulging in the short-term positive feelings that self-pity and other-pity often bring is easy, but if you do this be aware that you will perpetuate your tendency to feel hurt, and as such you will strengthen the irrational beliefs that underpin your hurt feelings.

You are more likely to refrain from seeking such sympathy if you are committed to feeling sorrow rather than hurt about being mistreated by others. If you are thus committed, then you will incorporate the rational beliefs that underpin sorrow when you tell other people what has happened to you.

Let me illustrate what I mean. What follows is how Susan talked about being badly treated by a friend, Cynthia, to another friend, Linda, first from the perspective of hurt-based, 'poor me' irrational beliefs and then as she would have talked about her feelings if she had held sorrow-based rational beliefs. Note how the dialogue proceeds differently.

Dialogue 1: Hurt-based

>*Susan (holding irrational beliefs):* I asked Cynthia to babysit for me and she said that she couldn't because she had to stay in and study. I then found out she had gone out with some of her friends and did not stay in at all. I always agree to babysit for her and this is the first time I have asked her to return the favour. She really should have returned the favour.
>
>*Linda:* Yes, I agree. She sounds very selfish.
>
>*Susan:* She is. I go out of my way to help her out and it's terrible that she not only refuses to help me, but lies to me as well.
>
>*Linda:* Poor you. You shouldn't be so good to her. She doesn't deserve to be your friend.
>
>*Susan:* That's what I think. I just like to be helpful and don't expect much in return.

In this interchange, note how Susan states her irrational belief when she tells Linda about Cynthia's behaviour ('She really should have returned the favour'). This leads Linda to respond that Cynthia is selfish, a rating of the whole of Cynthia with which Susan agrees. Susan then articulates another irrational belief ('... it's terrible that she not only refuses to help me, but lies to me as well'). Linda then overtly pities Susan ('Poor you'), to which Susan responds with more self-pity. This interchange shows the effect of 'poor me' irrational beliefs when left unchallenged.

Dialogue 2: Sorrow-based

>*Susan (holding rational beliefs):* I asked Cynthia to babysit for me and she said that she couldn't because she had to stay in and study. I then found out she had gone out with some of her friends and did not stay in at all. I always agree to babysit for

her and this is the first time I have asked her to return the favour. It would have been nice if she could have returned the favour, but she doesn't have to do so. However, I am a bit sorrowful and fed up about it, so I am going to tell her how I feel.

Linda: I would have felt hurt if I was you. She sounds very selfish.

Susan: She seems to have acted selfishly on this occasion, but I am sure she also acts non-selfishly at times. It's true that I have gone out of my way to help her out and it's a pain that she didn't return the compliment and seems to have lied to me, but hardly the end of the world.

Linda: Don't you feel sorry for yourself? If I were you, I would think that I shouldn't have been so good to her and that she doesn't deserve to be my friend.

Susan: I feel sorrowful that she hasn't helped out, but I don't feel sorry for myself. It's not a question, in my mind, of deservingness. It's a question of her not acting like a friend, and that is something that I am going to talk to her about.

Note how, in this interchange, Susan not only articulates rational beliefs when telling Linda about Cynthia's behaviour, but gently corrects Linda's own irrational beliefs. Also note how Susan refuses to feel sorry for herself throughout this interchange.

Consequently, if you want to feel sorrowful and not hurt, don't just strive to hold sorrow-based rational beliefs but, when you talk to people about how others have treated you badly, correct their irrational beliefs and resist the temptation to play the victim when they feel sorry for you.

Give up gain 2: Don't look to others to validate your hurt experience

As discussed in Chapter 2, when you feel hurt you tend to think that you have been badly treated by a person or people who are important to you, and you also think that you have done nothing to deserve such mistreatment. As I stressed in that chapter, it is not the inferences of mistreatment and undeservingness on their own that lead to your hurt feelings, but the irrational beliefs that you hold about such inferences that are the determining factor of your hurt.

Now, when you hold such irrational beliefs you tend to think that these inferences are true. In other words, you are in no doubt that you have been badly treated and that you do not deserve such mistreatment. As such, when you feel hurt and you tell others about how badly you were treated and how you have done nothing to deserve such behaviour, what you are looking for is validation of your experience. You want the person to whom you are talking to agree with you (1) that you have been badly treated; (2) that you don't deserve such treatment; and (3) that you are right to feel hurt. Conversely, you do not want the other person to question any of these three components. If they do, you may well feel hurt about their questioning! As such, you may seek out those people who are likely to validate your experience and keep away from those who are likely to question it.

So if you wish to become less prone to feeling hurt, apart from thinking rationally about the way others have treated you, refrain from seeking validation of your experience. Question for yourself whether others have treated you badly and whether you have wittingly or unwittingly contributed to the way they have treated you, and seek out others who may help you to question these aspects of your experience.

Give up gain 3: Stop complaining

When you tell people about how hurt you feel about your undeserved treatment at the hands of others, you are not only seeking sympathy and validation of your experience but are also engaging in the short-term pleasure of complaining, or what some people unkindly but perhaps accurately call 'whining'! Why complaining is enjoyable may be a mystery to some people, but if you engage in it a lot then face up to the possibility that you may find the very act of complaining enjoyable, irrespective of what it is designed to elicit from others.

Complaining, itself, gives you an opportunity to rehearse your irrational beliefs. Since complaining, when you feel hurt, is often underpinned by an awfulizing belief, every time you complain about the mistreatment you have received at the hands of others you are practising this irrational belief. So while stopping complaining will mean that you forego any short-term pleasure that you may derive from this activity, it will help you in the longer term because you will not be strengthening your hurt-based irrational beliefs, and you can use your time instead to challenge your irrational beliefs and strengthen your sorrow-based rational beliefs.

So if you wish to become less prone to feeling hurt when you discuss your experiences of being mistreated by others, do so from the perspective of your sorrow-based rational beliefs, and do so without complaint.

Learn about the familiarity principle and strive to go against it

The familiarity principle describes a tendency for humans to think, feel and act in ways that are familiar to them and to seek out situations that are familiar to them as well. Thus, if you are prone to hurt you will find the feelings, thoughts and behaviours that are involved in your hurt problem familiar and very easy to experience, even though they are detrimental to your well-being. Thus, in order for you to become less prone to hurt, you will need to tolerate the discomfort of holding sorrow-based rational beliefs and acting and thinking in ways that are consistent with them.

Please accept the discomfort that is almost always associated with personal change, and if you find yourself setting up situations that make it likely that you will experience your old familiar feelings of hurt, realize that you are operating according to the familiarity principle.

Understanding and learning from what you are doing, and renewing your resolve to tolerate the unfamiliarity of personal change, will help you to transcend the familiarity principle until you become used to experiencing sorrow and not hurt when you have truly been mistreated by others. In doing so you will become less prone to feeling hurt.

16

Question your role in others' mistreatment of you

So far in this part of the book, I have used the example of being mistreated in showing you how to make yourself less prone to feeling hurt. I just want to remind you that I am fully aware that you may feel hurt about different aspects of others' behaviour – as I discussed in Chapter 2. In this chapter, I will continue to use 'being mistreated' as an example, and will leave to you to apply what I have to say to what you are hurt about.

Now, I am going to ask you to consider the possibility that you have some role, albeit an unwitting one, in others' mistreatment of you. If this is the case then you may be helping to produce the very mistreatment about which you are prone to feel hurt.

'Me,' I hear you saying, 'training people to mistreat me? Why would you say that? Do you think that I am some kind of masochist? Do you think that I actually enjoy being mistreated? Not at all, I hate it. It's one of the last things in the world I want to happen to me.'

Lack of protest

I fully understand that being mistreated is one of the last things in the world that you want to happen to you, but let me put it this way. When you feel hurt about being mistreated, do you promptly go up to the person who has mistreated you and indicate your displeasure in a way that is clear, non-blaming and indicates to the other person that whatever he or she may think, in your view you have been mistreated and you want such behaviour to cease?

The chances are that if you are hurt about being mistreated, you do no such thing. Indeed, you tend to do the exact opposite. You tend to avoid the other person, or if you do not physically avoid him (in this case) you emotionally withdraw from him. Either way, the person who has, in your view, mistreated you, in all probability does not know how you feel.

If the person does not know how you feel, then the following are possible:

- The person does not consider that he has mistreated you.
- The person may read your silence as indicating that you do not think that you have been mistreated. After all, you did not complain!
- The person may read your silence as indicating that while you think you have been mistreated, you don't mind such treatment. After all, once again you did not complain!
- The person has no thoughts about the incident at all.

If any of the above is the case, the consequence is that the person may well continue you to treat you in the same manner. He will do so because you have done nothing to discourage him from doing so. As my friend and colleague Dr Paul Hauck has often said:

> You get the behaviour from others that you put up with without protest.

So, by not saying anything to the person who has mistreated you, you may be unwittingly training him to mistreat you in future.

It is important, therefore, that you assert yourself with the person who has mistreated you, particularly when it is clear that you have been badly treated. Indeed, it is important that you do so promptly. If the person knows how you feel and knows about this very soon after his behaviour towards you, he will be challenged to think about his behaviour. Even if he rationalizes it to himself and with you, at least he knows that you are not prepared to tolerate such behaviour in the future, and so he is less likely to mistreat you.

If you would like to know more about how to assert yourself, the obstacles to such assertion and how to address these obstacles effectively, consult the book that I wrote with my colleague Daniel Constantinou for Sheldon Press, *Assertiveness Step by Step* (2004).

Aggression

Another way that you may unwittingly get more mistreatment from others is to be aggressive towards them when they have mistreated you, or when you think that they have mistreated you. This applies when there is a strong unhealthy angry component to your hurt. When you are aggressive towards the person who has mistreated you, you will usually be verbally aggressive towards them or you will act in an aggressive way towards them. The trouble with aggression is that it begets aggression.

So, when someone mistreats you and you are aggressive towards them, they will consider that you have mistreated them and respond in kind. In this way, your aggressive response to the original mistreatment ends up helping to create more mistreatment of you.

In order to break this cycle, you need to do two things.

First, you need to challenge the irrational beliefs that underpin your feelings of unhealthy anger linked to your hurt feelings. Look for and challenge your demand and the other depreciation belief that stems from your demand.

Second, instead of acting aggressively to the person who has mistreated you, use assertion to indicate your healthy annoyance about the way you have been treated and seek an agreement from the person that he or she will not mistreat you in future.

Treating others too well

You may think that if you treat people well, then they are likely to treat you well in return, and with certain exceptions you would be right. However, if you treat people too well, if you are too generous towards them, then two things may happen. First, the other people may reciprocate but without matching your generosity. Consequently, you may consider their response as mistreatment because they have treated you less well than you have treated them.

Second, the other people may avoid you after you have been over-generous towards them. Yes, that's right – when others are in receipt of your excessive generosity, they may avoid you. Why might this be the case?

First, the other person may not want your extreme generosity. She (in this case) may see it as an obligation to respond in kind, and she may resent this obligation. To get out of this obligation she avoids you.

Second, the other person may want to respond to your extreme generosity, but is unable to do so. If she meets you and fails to respond in kind, she is likely to feel ashamed of her failure to match your generosity, and therefore to stop herself from feeling ashamed she avoids you.

Whether the person responds to your extreme generosity with lesser generosity or with avoidance, you may see both responses as mistreatment of you. However, by being over-generous you have played an active role in contributing to the other's behaviour. If you do often feel hurt about being badly treated by others because they have failed to respond in kind to your generous behaviour, it is important that you first deal with your hurt feelings, by addressing and changing your irrational beliefs. Then you need to consider the level of your generosity towards others and do one of two things:

- Scale back your generosity to levels where people feel able to respond in kind.
- Keep being over-generous towards others, but stop demanding that people have to respond in kind or, indeed, at all!

17

Check for your biases concerning others' behaviour

You will recall that in Chapter 2 I discussed how we tend to feel hurt when we make one or more inferences about what people who are significant have done to us, or about what they have failed to do. Table 4 provides a summary of this material.

Inferences about what others have done	Inferences about what others have not done
Criticized me unfairly	Neglected me
Rejected me	Unfairly excluded me
Disapproved of me	Failed to appreciate me
Betrayed me	Deprived me of what I deserved
Used me	

Table 4 Inferences about what others have either done or not done when we experience hurt

As I also discussed in Chapter 2, if you are prone to feeling hurt, it is likely that you hold one or more general irrational beliefs. These general irrational beliefs have a biasing effect on what you pay attention to in your relationships and the inferences that you make about what others have done or failed to do.

Let's take the case of Veronica. Veronica is prone to hurt, and the theme that keeps recurring in her description of what happens to her that she feels hurt about is that she thinks her friends do not appreciate her. When she actually feels hurt in specific situations, she is convinced that her friends have not shown her due appreciation. As I discussed throughout Part 2 of this book, when Veronica is actually experiencing hurt feelings in a given situation, she needs to assume temporarily that her inference at 'A' is correct in that situation (i.e. it was true that her friends did not show her appreciation) and then she needs to identify, question and change the specific irrational belief that underpins her hurt feelings. She is then in a position to go back to 'A' and question its validity.

Doing this will help Veronica to question the specific inferences that she makes at 'A' in specific hurt episodes, but if she is particularly prone to feel hurt about lack of appreciation in general then she needs to do something else. Let's see what Veronica actually did with help from her counsellor.

1 First, Veronica acknowledged that when she feels hurt, she tends to feel hurt about her friends not showing her due appreciation. She arrived at this conclusion by thinking about her past episodes of hurt and by asking herself what she tends to feel hurt about. However, she could also have arrived at this conclusion by formally assessing her specific hurt episodes as recommended in Part 2 of this book.

2 Veronica then recognized that her general hurt-related irrational belief – 'People must show me appreciation every time I have done something nice for them' – had a biasing effect on what she paid attention to in her relationships with friends. She realized that when she did something nice for her friends she was always checking her answerphone messages and her text messages to see whether or not they had contacted her to say thank you. She also realized that after she had done something nice for her friends, she had recurring images of them showing her appreciation.

3 Veronica realized that if her friends had not contacted her very soon after she had done something nice for them, she quickly assumed that their silence meant that they did not appreciate her. She saw with clarity that her general irrational belief had a biasing effect on the inferences that she made about their attitude to her. In a similar vein, Veronica saw that even when her friends did say thank you for what she had done for them, she still inferred that they did not appreciate her if, in her view, their 'thank you' was not sufficiently fulsome.

4 With help from her therapist, Veronica saw that because she held rigid ideas about being appreciated, she did not take into account that others could show her appreciation but do so in their own way and in their own time frame. In order for her

to 'feel' appreciated, therefore, Veronica first viewed the matter from the perspective of her general rational belief (i.e. 'I want people to show me appreciation every time I do something nice for them, but really they do not have to do so'). Then she trained herself to accept her friends' messages of appreciation even when they were often less fulsome than her own, and even when they took much longer to show appreciation than she did when they did something nice for her.

5 Veronica learned, in effect, that people were different when it came to showing appreciation. Most took much longer than she did to show appreciation, and most were less fulsome in their appreciative comments than she was.

6 Finally, with help from her therapist, Veronica decided that if a particular friend had not shown any appreciation a week after she had done something nice for them, then she would express both sorrow to her friend and her preference for receiving such appreciation. She also agreed that in the intervening time period she would not check her answerphone or her mobile for messages of appreciation from the friend. She further resolved that she would accept, but not engage with, any residual thinking about her friend not showing her appreciation that persisted after she periodically challenged her general irrational beliefs.

Veronica became less prone to hurt about friends not showing her due appreciation, partly because she operated largely on her general rational beliefs about not being appreciated, but partly because she corrected her biases about receiving such appreciation.

Correcting biases in viewing and making inferences about others' behaviour

Let me outline some general principles that you can follow when correcting your own hurt-related biases in viewing and making inferences about others' behaviour. In doing so, I suggest that you refer back to the example of Veronica.

1 Write down what you feel mainly hurt about (see Table 4 for assistance). This theme will also be apparent from the specific examples of your hurt.

2 Write down your major hurt-related general irrational belief.

3 Write down how this belief may bias
   (a)   what you pay attention to with respect to others' behaviour when you feel hurt; and
   (b)   what inferences you make about others' behaviour in such circumstances.

4 Challenge your general irrational belief and rehearse the rational alternative to this belief.

5 From this general rational belief, consider alternative inferences and focus on aspects of the situations you may have neglected (use the questions presented on p. 83).

6 Allow sufficient time to pass before concluding that your hurt-related inference is proven true on the basis of probability, and then assert yourself with the person concerned.

18

Understand others from their perspective

So far in this part of the book, I have suggested that you do the following in order to become less prone to feeling hurt:

- Acknowledge that hurt is a problem for you and prepare to change.
- Develop general sorrow-based rational beliefs.
- Think and act in ways that are consistent with your general rational beliefs.
- Question your role in others' mistreatment of you.
- Check for your biases in viewing and making inferences about others' behaviour.

Once you have taken the above steps, you are ready to understand the behaviour of the person you hitherto thought had mistreated you. In her famous book *To Kill a Mockingbird*, one of Harper Lee's characters says that you can only understand someone once you have walked a mile in their moccasins. Counsellors call this type of understanding *empathic understanding*.

In order to understand the behaviour of the person who in your view has mistreated you, you need to:

1 think rationally and be free from hurt; and
2 be motivated to understand the other person's behaviour.

Assuming that you have met the above two conditions, this is what you need to do:

1 Approach the person you consider has mistreated you and ask her (in this case) if you can discuss something with her.
2 If she agrees, describe her behaviour that you now feel sorrowful about and 'own' your feelings. It is very important that you are descriptive in your account: don't make inferences about

her behaviour. For example, say, 'I felt sorrowful that you did not say thank you when I loaned you £100' rather than 'You mistreated me by ignoring me when I loaned you £100.' Note that the former uses only descriptive language while the latter uses inferential and pejorative language. The other person is likely to respond healthily to the former and defensively to the latter. Also say 'I felt sorrowful when you . . .' rather than 'You made me feel ...'

3 Ask the person for her response. If she agrees with your view, tell her that you would really like to understand her behaviour. If she disagrees with you, ask her to tell you what happened from her point of view.

4 Proceed until the other person considers that you understand her from her perspective.

5 Once you have understood the other person from her perspective you can respond to her accordingly. If you agree with her account, for example, you might revise your view that you were mistreated and proceed with your relationship accordingly. If you disagree with her account, explain to her why you disagree and suggest that you both agree to differ. If she agrees to differ, then you can proceed with your relationship more or less intact. If she refuses to agree to differ, then your relationship may be threatened and it may be worth suggesting to her that you should both sleep on the matter and discuss it at an agreed later date.

19

Develop and rehearse a healthy philosophy of relationships

In my book *How to Make Yourself Miserable* (Sheldon Press, 2001), I showed that when you are prone to hurt you operate on a view of the world that is founded on the irrational beliefs that underpin this emotion. I discussed the elements of this world view, and how they influence the inferences that you make, in Chapter 2. Consequently, in order to become less prone to hurt it is important that you develop a world view founded on sorrow-related rational beliefs. I outlined such a world view in Chapter 3, but let me elaborate on what I said then.

The following are what I said in Chapter 3 were the major components of the sorrow-based world view:

- *World view:* When I do a lot for people, most will reciprocate, but some will not.
- *World view:* I will not betray the trust of those close to me and they will usually not betray me, although a minority will.
- *World view:* I will be fair to significant others and they will in the main be fair to me, although a few won't.
- *World view:* Those close to me may exclude me or neglect me for no good reason, but will do so only rarely.

If you look at these world views carefully, you will see that there is one theme that unites them. It is the theme of exceptions. No matter how well you treat people and no matter how many will reciprocate, there will be exceptions. This may be seen as a healthy philosophy of relationships or the rational version of the golden rule:

Treat people well and they will normally treat you well, but not inevitably so. This rule applies even with people to whom you are very, very close.

Thus, if you want to become less prone to hurt, you do need to embrace the idea that those with whom you are in relation are ultimately fallible human beings who are guided by what is in their heads, not by how much you have done for them. Accept this reality and you will certainly feel sorrow when you are mistreated, but you will not feel hurt in any enduring sense.

You may see the sense of this but think that while this applies to others' lives it does not or should not apply to you. If you do believe this, re-read the section on personal immunity on pp. 96–7.

Identify what really matters in your relationships and actively develop these factors

If you fully appreciate that all your relationships are guided by the rational golden rule as discussed above, you will accept this as an unfortunate feature of relationships that cannot be eradicated. This realization will help you to discover what really matters in your relationships. I am not going to speculate on what that is, and it is certainly not my place to outline what that should be. Rather, I want to make the point that when you are less prone to hurt you will be able to look at your relationships from a broad perspective and discover and pursue what is important about relationships for you as a unique individual.

I have now come to the end of this book. I hope you have found it useful. If you would like to give me feedback on it and how you have applied it to your problems with hurt, I would be glad to hear from you. Please write to me c/o Sheldon Press.

Index